Engels voor zorg en welzijn

Engels voor zorg en welzijn
Niveau 4

Ank van de Wiel

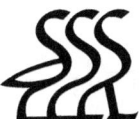

Bohn Stafleu van Loghum
Houten 2007

© Bohn Stafleu van Loghum, 2007

Alle rechten voorbehouden. Niets uit deze uitgave mag worden verveelvoudigd, opgeslagen in een geautomatiseerd gegevensbestand, of openbaar gemaakt, in enige vorm of op enige wijze, hetzij elektronisch, mechanisch, door fotokopieën of opnamen, hetzij op enige andere manier, zonder voorafgaande schriftelijke toestemming van de uitgever.

Voor zover het maken van kopieën uit deze uitgave is toegestaan op grond van artikel 16b Auteurswet 1912 j° het Besluit van 20 juni 1974, Stb. 351, zoals gewijzigd bij het Besluit van 23 augustus 1985, Stb. 471 en artikel 17 Auteurswet 1912, dient men de daarvoor wettelijk verschuldigde vergoedingen te voldoen aan de Stichting Reprorecht (Postbus 3051, 2130 KB Hoofddorp). Voor het overnemen van (een) gedeelte(n) uit deze uitgave in bloemlezingen, readers en andere compilatiewerken (artikel 16 Auteurswet 1912) dient men zich tot de uitgever te wenden.

Samensteller(s) en uitgever zijn zich volledig bewust van hun taak een betrouwbare uitgave te verzorgen. Niettemin kunnen zij geen aansprakelijkheid aanvaarden voor drukfouten en andere onjuistheden die eventueel in deze uitgave voorkomen.

ISBN 978 90 313 4987 6
NUR 897, 632

Ontwerp omslag: A-Graphics Design, Apeldoorn
Ontwerp binnenwerk: Studio Bassa, Culemborg
Automatische opmaak: Pre Press, Zeist
Cartoons: Studio Imago, Apeldoorn
Foto's: Hollandse Hoogte, Amsterdam

Bohn Stafleu van Loghum
Het Spoor 2
Postbus 246
3990 GA Houten

www.bsl.nl

Distributeur in België:
Standaard Uitgeverij
Mechelsesteenweg 203
2018 Antwerpen

www.standaarduitgeverij.be

Wat staat er in het boek?

In dit boek komen vreemde taal, beroep en burgerschap samen tot een logisch geheel.

Voor studenten in de zorg- en welzijnssector neemt taal een centrale plaats in. Niet alleen in maatschappelijke maar ook in beroepssituaties is taal een belangrijk instrument om te kunnen functioneren.

De maatschappij waarin studenten leven en werken is veranderd. Er wordt van hen verwacht dat ze hun rol als burger serieus nemen. Burgerschap gaat over je eigen mening leren geven, het ontwikkelen van een bewuste en kritische houding, oefenen om voor jezelf en je beroep op te komen. Een respectvolle (beroeps)houding is terug te vinden in alle burgerschapselementen. In dit boek wordt daarom steeds de link gemaakt beroep, maatschappij en de taal die hierbij het instrument is.

De ontwikkelingen op de werkvloer hebben ook niet stil gestaan. Op het werk worden cliënten steeds mondiger en de problemen die ze hebben complexer. Er wordt een groot beroep gedaan op sociale en communicatieve vaardigheden. Een goede beroepshouding is een voorwaarde voor succes.

Veel eisen die in burgerschap geformuleerd zijn, zijn niet alleen relevant maar vaak onmisbaar voor deze beroepsgroepen. Algemene competenties als samenwerken, aandacht en begrip tonen, ethisch en integer handelen en omgaan met druk en tegenslag vormen het hart van het beroep. Deze competenties komen dan ook veelvuldig aan bod. Het beroep speelt zich niet alleen meer binnen de landsgrenzen af. Vanuit de eigen multiculturele samenleving kijken studenten steeds vaker verder dan hun eigen land. Buitenlandse stages en Engelstalige informatie op internet of vakliteratuur is niet meer weg te denken uit de opleiding.

SPECIFIEKE INVULLING VAN HET BOEK

- Persoonlijke ontwikkeling en ontwikkeling van beroepshouding staan centraal.
- De student ontwikkelt taalvaardigheden door te oefenen met beroepssituaties.
- De taalinhoud dekt de eisen uit het raamwerk moderne vreemde talen (MVT) in het secundair onderwijs.
- De inhoud dekt de eisen van het brondocument Leren, Loopbaan en Burgerschap.
- Ieder hoofdstuk gaat over een kerntaak uit het brondocument Leren, Loopbaan en Burgerschap. Een kerntaak is vertaald naar een beroepsgerichte inhoud, zoals het sturen van de eigen loopbaan of collegiaal opstellen.
- De student ontwikkelt per kerntaak een aantal algemene competenties zoals vakdeskundigheid toepassen, presenteren of analyseren.

OPBOUW

Iedere hoofdstuk van het boek heeft een vaste structuur. Soms zijn er extra oefeningen voor spreekvaardigheid of grammatica ingevoegd.
- Het hoofdstuk begint met een pittige leestekst met vragen.
- Hierna volgt een luisteroefening die op de bijgeleverde cd te beluisteren is.
- Het derde onderdeel bestaat uit verschillende grammaticaoefeningen.

- De schrijfvaardigheid komt steeds in de tweede helft van het hoofdstuk aan bod. Onderzoeksopdrachten zijn op verschillende plaatsen toegevoegd. In deze opdrachten wordt steeds gebruikgemaakt van het internet.

Overzicht algemene competenties in de zes units.

		unit 1	unit 2	unit 3	unit 4	unit 5	unit 6
a	beslissen en activiteiten initiëren	×	×	×	×	×	×
b	aansturen	×	×	×			
c	begeleiden	×	×	×			
d	aandacht en begrip tonen	×	×			×	
e	samenwerken en overleggen	×	×	×	×	×	×
f	ethisch en integer handelen	×		×		×	×
g	relaties bouwen en netwerken	×					
h	overtuigen en beïnvloeden	×	×	×	×	×	
i	presenteren	×	×			×	
j	formuleren en rapporteren	×	×		×	×	
k	vakdeskundigheid toepassen	×		×			×
l	materialen en middelen inzetten	×	×				×
m	analyseren	×	×		×	×	×
n	onderzoeken	×	×	×	×	×	×
o	creëren en innoveren		×				
p	leren	×	×	×	×	×	
q	plannen en organiseren		×				
r	op de behoeften en verwachtingen van de 'klant' richten				×		
s	kwaliteit leveren	×	×	×		×	
t	instructies en procedures opvolgen		×	×	×	×	×
u	omgaan met verandering en aanpassen	×		×			
v	met druk en tegenslag omgaan		×	×			
w	gedrevenheid en ambitie tonen	×	×				
x	ondernemend en commercieel handelen	×					×
y	bedrijfsmatig handelen						×

Inhoud

1	**How to survive my career**	13
1.1	Reading	13
	What do you do?	13
	Questions about the text	14
1.2	Listening Skills 1	16
	How to behave?	16
	Idioms	17
1.3	Research	18
	A. Code of conduct for nurses	18
	B. Code of Practice for Social Care Workers	18
	Exercise	19
1.4	Grammar: the (Simple) Present Tense (tegenwoordige tijd)	19
	Grammar: the Simple Present tense	20
1.5	Translation	20
1.6	Writing	21
	Job application	21
1.7	Speaking	23
	Job interview	23
	Role play	24
1.8	Grammar: Prepositions	24
	Exercise	24
1.9	Research and Conversation	24
	Networking	24
1.10	Speaking	25
	Presentation: improve the quality of your work	25
1.11	Grammar: the Present Continuous Tense	25
	Grammar: the Present Continuous Tense	26
	Grammar: the Simple Present Tense of the Present Continuous Tense	26
1.12	Reading and research	27
	Finding the right job	27
2	**How to survive my beliefs**	29
2.1	Reading	29
	Young people need strong voice	29
	Questions about the text	30
2.2	Research	31
	Europe on the Internet	31
2.3	Listening Skills 2	33
	Ten reasons for joining a union	33
	Idioms	34
	Extra questions	35
2.4	Grammar: the (Simple) Past Tense (verleden tijd)	35

	Grammar: the Past Tense	36
2.5	Word Combinations	36
	Exercise	36
2.6	Speaking	36
	Role play: I Want change	36
2.7	Listening Skills 3	37
	Vote for me!	37
	Exercise	38
	Extra questions	38
2.8	Translation	39
	Exercise	39
2.9	Write your own campaign or party programme	39
2.10	Reading	40
	A Window on Europe: what do you think?	40
	Idioms	41
	Extra questions	42
2.11	Speaking	42
	What to do if people don't treat you right?	42
3	**How to survive my organization**	**45**
3.1	Reading	45
	Too many young people are getting hurt at work	45
	Questions about the text	46
3.2	Listening Skill 4	47
	Performance interview	47
	Idioms	48
3.3	Conversation	49
	When things go wrong	49
	Social worker removed from register after misconduct found	49
	Tips voor de discussieleider	50
	Helpful phrases to use in the discussion	50
3.4	Grammar: the Future Tense (toekomende tijd)	51
	Grammar: the Future Tense	52
3.5	Translation	52
	Exercise	52
3.6	Listening Skills 5	53
	Can you help us?	54
	Exercise	55
3.7	Fluency: How to give advice	55
	Exercise	56
3.8	Grammar: Much, many, little, few	57
	Exercise	57
3.9	Writing	57
	Happy at work	57
3.11	Grammar: a or an	58
	Exercise	58
3.12	Conversation	58
	Coaching	58
4	**How to survive my shopping?**	**61**
4.1	How to choose a mobile service	61
	Mobile services	61
	Questions about the text	63
4.2	Listening Skills 6	64
	Idioms	65

4.3	Research	65
	Shopping on the Internet	65
	Assignment	65
4.4	Grammar: Questions and negations	66
	Exercise	67
4.5	Translation	68
	Exercise	68
4.6	Writing	69
	Product information	69
4.7	Speaking	69
4.8	Reading	70
	Are you in debt?	70
	Exercise	71
4.9	Grammar: Personal and Possessive Pronouns	72
	Exercise	73
4.10	Writing	73
	Numbers	73
5	**How to survive my norms and values?**	**75**
5.1	Reading	75
	Do we need citizenship?	75
	Questions about the text	76
5.2	Listening Skills 7	77
	Private and professional attitude	77
	Idioms	78
5.3	Speaking	79
5.4	Grammar: the Present Perfect Tense	80
	Exercise	81
5.5	Translation	81
	Exercise	81
5.6	Writing	82
	Program for exchange students	82
	Exercise	82
5.7	Reading and research	83
	About Amnesty International	83
	5.8 Listening Skills 8	84
	Flight from Vietnam	84
	Idioms	85
5.9	Grammar: Relative Pronouns	86
	Exercise	87
5.10	Conversation	87
	Exercise	87
6	**How to survive?**	**89**
6.1	Reading	89
	Keeping yourself healthy	89
	Questions about the text	91
6.2	Listening Skills 9	92
	Healthier life	92
	Idioms	93
6.3	Speaking and research	94
	Advice on health and safety by the telephone	94
6.4	Grammar: Adjectives and Adverbs	95
	Exercise	95
6.5	Research and Writing	96

	Sexual health	96
	Exercise	96
6.6	Reading and research	97
	Anatomy	97
6.7	Grammar	98
	The Plural	98
	Exercise	99
6.8	Idioms	99
	Exercise	99
6.9	Writing and Conversation	100
	Healthy way of life	100
6.10	Reading	101
	State of mind: What keeps people mentally well?	101
	Exercise	102

Appendix A — 103
Irregular verbs (onregelmatige werkwoorden) — 103

Appendix B — 105
Vocabulary English – Dutch — 105

Key — 125
Unit 1 — 125
1.1 Questions about the text — 125
1.2 How to behave? Idioms — 125
1.3 Research — 125
1.4 Grammar: the Present Tense — 126
1.5 Translation — 127
1.8 Prepositions — 127
1.11 Grammar — 127
Unit 2 — 128
2.1 Young people need strong voice — 128
2.3 Listening Skill 2 — 128
2.4 Grammar: The Past Tense — 129
2.5 Verbs — 129
2.7 Listening Skill 3 — 129
2.8 Translation — 130
2.10 A window on Europe: what do you think? — 130
Unit 3 — 130
3.1 Too many young people are getting hurt at work — 130
3.2 Performance interview — 130
3.4 Grammar: The Future Tense — 131
3.5 Translation — 131
3.6 Listening Skill 5 — 131
3.8 Grammar: much, many, little, few — 132
3.10 Grammar: A or an — 132
Unit 4 — 132
4.1 How to choose a mobile service — 132
4.2 I have been robbed! — 132
4.4 Grammar: Questions and Negations — 133
4.5 Translation — 133
4.8 Reading — 134
4.9 Grammar: Personal and Possessive Pronouns — 134
4.10 Writing — 134
Unit 5 — 135

5.1 Do we need Citizenship?	135
5.2 Private and professional attitude	135
5.4 Grammar: The Present Perfect Tense	136
5.5 Translation	136
5.8 Flight from Vietnam	136
5.9 Grammar: Relative Pronouns	136
Unit 6	137
6.1 Food and health	137
6.2 Healthier life	137
6.4 Grammar: Adjectives and Adverbs	138
6.6 Anatomy	138
6.7 The Plural	138
6.8 Idioms	139
6.10 State of mind	139

1 How to survive my career

1.1 Reading

Read the following text.

Foto: Felix Kalkman/
Hollandse Hoogte

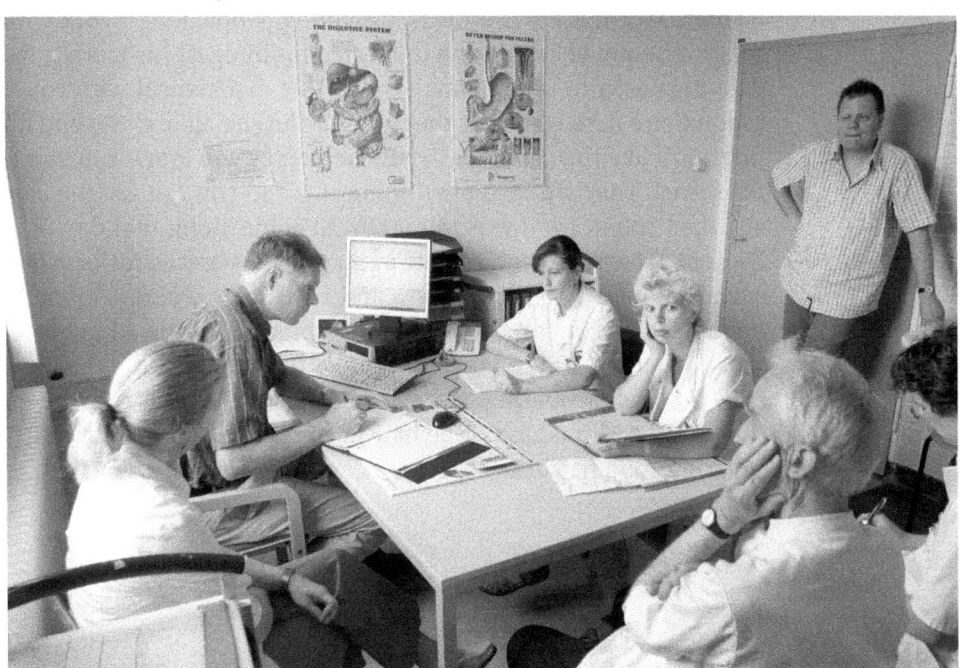

What do you do?

When you are still at school it is difficult to know exactly where or in which field you want to work. [According to] an [advertisement] nurses:
- [enjoy] working with people;
- are interested in [disease] prevention and health promotion;
- like to [provide] [care] to those who are [ill] or injured;
- are interested in providing or influencing health care by working with members of the [community], health care professionals and [policy makers].

It may sound interesting but what is nursing like in the real world? This does [of course] depend on the sort of nursing you choose to do. Are you going to work with children, do you prefer the care of the elderly or is [mental nursing] your thing? Whatever you choose the [focus of attention] for a qualified nurse is the patient. It is [not simply] the [condition] from which he or she may be [suffering], but also the [needs] and [anxieties] that are caused by the condition. This [includes] the [pressures] on family and friends. Your place of work may be a hospital [ward] or specialist clinic, or it could be out in the [community] – visiting people at home or [attached] to local [health centres]. Nurses are playing an [increasingly] [prominent] role in the [provision] of [health care] in the community.

So what does a social care worker do? A social care worker looks after the health and [welfare] of the [population]. We are all [likely] to [become] clients of [social care services] [at one time] or another but some of the main groups include children or families who are under stress, people with [disabilities], people with emotional or [psychological] [difficulties], people with financial or [housing problems] and older people who need help with [daily living activities].

Social care services [deal with] many [issues] and so they can [operate] in many [settings]. Social care services may be [offered] in hospitals or health centres, in [educational settings], in community groups, in [residential homes], in advice centres or even in people's own homes.

This is how one sociale worker describes her work: 'Most of the people that I work with are 18. When I meet them it is the first time that they are leaving [foster placements]. My [primary task] with the young people that I work with is helping them to set up a home, helping them to be able to [budget] [properly], that type of thing. You definitely need to bring some of your [life experience] with you to this job. [Qualifications] are important but they are not the [be all and the end all]. When you come into a job like this, and you see those people you know you can make a difference to their lives. They are [actually] [grateful], and you can see the emotion on their face and then you know it was important to come along that day.'

Because there is a strong focus in the health services for organisations and professionals to work together, nurses and social care workers often [meet]. When, for example, a person is coming out of hospital following a hip operation, he may need a [host] of other care to [ensure] that he [recovers] well in his own home and [maintain] his [independence]. As well as [ongoing] health care, he may need help with [dressing] and washing or he may need special [equipment] such as [grab rails] or a [walking frame]. These aspects of care would all be [arranged] by social services departments.

Questions about the text

1. *injured* in line 5 stands for:
a insecure
b cured
c damaged or impaired
d mentally handicapped

2. *depend on* in line 10 stands for:
a is represented by
b is looked after by
c wanted by
d is determined by

3. *qualified* in line 12 means:
a someone who has passed the final exam
b someone who is still a student
c someone who is at university
d someone who is emphatic

4. *the focus of attention* in line 12 means:
a the things they see

b the things they want to do
c the things they don't do
d the main thing they do

5. A [qualified] nurse:
a has [passed] her exams.
b has [failed] her exams.
c cannot [apply] for a job.
d can only work with adults.

6. *in the [community]* in line 16 refers to:
a in the clinic
b [in the country]
c in the hospital
d at people's own home

7. One of the tasks of a social care worker is:
a to wash people.
b to help people to look after themselves.
c to sing to people.
d to make [equipment] for people.

8. An example of a psychological difficulty is:
a not to be able to dress.
b to suffer from [diabetes].
c to be [cheerful].
d to suffer from depression.

9. A [homeless person] has:
a a [psychological difficulty].
b an illness.
c a housing problem.
d a [bad temper].

10. To work in [close] [partnership] means:
a to work closely together.
b to be close to each other.
c to [watch closely].
d to be married with someone.

11. *to [recover]* in line 41 means:
a to find
b to fall ill
c to become well again
d to [cover up]

12. *independence* in line 42 refers to:
a the [ability] to do your own thing
b [private care]
c living in hospital
d the ability [to boss someone around]

13. Grab rails are for:
a people who want to grab each other.
b trains.

c children who cannot walk.
d individuals who need [support] when standing or changing [position].

1.2
Listening Skills 1

How to behave?

In caring for patients and clients you are personally [accountable] for your actions. Most professions have a code of conduct. This code describes the professional conduct and skills that are [required] of care workers as they go about their [daily] routine.

Listen to the following [conversation] that two students (Jack (J) and Laura (L) have with a nurse Louise (Lo) and a social care worker Pete (P).

L: Louise, is it true that they have actually written down how you have [to behave] at work? I find that very [scary]. It's like someone is watching you all the time.

Lo: Well, that's a bit exaggerated. If you do your job [properly], then you have nothing to worry about.

J: Can you give me an example of a nurse who doesn't do her job properly?

Lo: Er... For example, if someone doesn't obtain [consent] before they provide treatment or care or if they do not [protect] confidential information or respect the patient or client as an individual.

L: You see, that are too many [examples] to remember already. What do they mean by respect, just being nice to someone?

Lo: Whenever you talk about a patient's details [loudly] so other people can [overhear] the information you are disrespectful of someone.

L: So this code only applies to patients or clients?

Lo: No, it doesn't. It also applies to [employers], your colleagues, anyone who uses the service and other [carers].

J: Pete, do you have such a code as well?

P: Yes, we have the Code of Practice for Social Care Workers. We are [responsible] for making sure that our conduct does not [fall below] the standards as [set out] in this code.

J: How do you mean fall below? Not sticking to the rules or something like that?

P: Yes, for example when you do not respect or observe the dignity and privacy of [service users]. When someone does not [adhere] to policies and procedures, for example where it concerns accepting [gifts].

Lo: Do you receive gifts as well?

P: Oh yeah, I remember this elderly lady who [insisted] on giving me her golden [necklace] with a very expensive stone in it. She was so upset when I did not accept her gift. She just could not understand why I did not take it. No one has to know, she kept saying.

L: What a [shame]. Sometimes I think the rules are too [strict].

Lo: Maybe they are, but what about [confused] people who give away their [belongings] and later forget all about it. Not to mention angry family members! You have to protect your clients.

J: So what about abuse or [neglect]? Have you ever [come across] anything like that? You hear such horror stories in the [press].

Lo: Well, [luckily], I haven't seen any of that with my colleagues. However, there were some child neglect and abuse cases that came through the [paediatric ward]. That was [horrible]!

L: How do you know for sure [whether] someone is being abused?

P: You always have to be very [careful] about that. Bruises are [usually] a good sign to go on.

L: And what if a client accuses you of neglect and you haven't done anything wrong?

P: Well, [according] to the Code of Conduct, your employer must protect you from this by providing information. This is what the written policies and procedures are used for. When the information or your training is not enough your employer should provide training to [strengthen] and [develop] your [skills] and [knowledge].

Lo: You should not [worry] about all this. If you just do your work properly and respectfully and use [common sense], you will [enjoy] it as much as we do!

idioms

Vertaal de volgende woorden uit het gesprek:

1. gedragscode –
2. overdreven –
3. zorgen maken –
4. behandeling –
5. vertrouwelijke informatie –
6. patiëntengegevens –
7. collega's –
8. waardigheid –
9. gedragslijnen –
10. ontvangen –
11. overstuur –
12. regels –
13. beschermen –
14. misbruik –
15. gruwelverhalen –
16. gevallen –
17. zeker weten –
18. blauwe plekken –
19. beschuldigt –
20. beschermen –

1.3 Research

A. [Code of conduct] for nurses

The purpose of the 'NMC[1] code of professional conduct', standards for conduct, [performance] and ethics is to:
- inform the professions of the standard of professional conduct [required] of them in the [exercise of] their professional [accountability] and [practice];
- inform the public, other professions and [employers] of the standard of professional conduct that they can [expect] of a [registered practitioner].

As a registered nurse you are personally accountable for your practice. In caring for patients and clients, you must:
- respect the patient or client as an individual;
- [obtain consent] before you give any treatment or care;
- protect [confidential information];
- co-operate with others in the team;
- [maintain] your professional [knowledge] and competence;
- be [trustworthy];
- act to [identify] and minimise risk to patients and clients.

B. [Code of Practice] for Social Care Workers

The [purpose] of this code is to [set out] the conduct that is expected of social care workers and to inform [service users] and the public about the standards of conduct they can expect from social care workers. It forms part of the wider [package] of [legislation], practice standards and employers' [policies and procedures] that social care workers must meet. Social care workers are responsible for making sure that their conduct does not [fall below] the standards set out in this code and that no action or [omission] on their part [harms] the [wellbeing] of service users.

Social care workers must:
- Protect the rights and [promote] the [interests] of service users and carers;
- [Strive] to [establish] and [maintain] the trust and confidence of service users and carers;
- Promote the [independence] of service users [while] protecting them as far as possible from danger or harm;
- Respect the rights of service users while [seeking] to ensure that their [behaviour] does not harm themselves or other people;
- [Uphold] public trust and confidence in social care services;
- Be [accountable] for the quality of their work and take [responsibility] for maintaining and [improving] their knowledge and [skills].

Find out more on: www.gscc.org.uk (codes of practice).

---

1 The Nursing and [Midwifery] [Council] is an organisation set up by Parliament to protect the public by [ensuring] that nurses and midwives [provide] high standards of care to their patients and clients. Find out more on: http://www.nmc-uk.org/(NMC Code of Conduct).

1 HOW TO SURVIVE MY CAREER

Exercise

Read one of the texts above A nurse or B social care worker and then try to answer the following questions:

1. What is the purpose of the code?

A

B

2. Two examples of the things a social care worker / nurse should do are:

3. Two examples of the things a social care worker / nurse should *not* do are:

4. What is your view on the use of a code of conduct?

1.4 Grammar: the (Simple) Present Tense (tegenwoordige tijd)

De *Simple Present Tense* wordt in de volgende gevallen gebruikt.

1. Als er iets in het heden gebeurt.

Today she works with Mary.	–	Vandaag werkt ze met Mary.
Mr Smith goes home.	–	Meneer Smith gaat naar huis.

2. Als iets herhaaldelijk of volgens een schema gebeurt.

We always give sound advise.	–	We geven altijd degelijk advies.
Every day the centre opens at 8 am.	–	Het centrum gaat elke dag om 8 uur open.

3. Als het om een feit gaat.

Water freezes at zero degrees Celsius.	–	Water bevriest bij nul graden Celsius.
She lives in a shelter for battered women.	–	Ze woont in een opvanghuis voor mishandelde vrouwen.

De *Present Tense* wordt gevormd door het **hele werkwoord**.

I *work* as a community worker.	–	Ik werk als opbouwwerker.

Na **he, she** of **it** krijg je het **hele werkwoord + (e)s**.

John *visits* his clients in the morning.	–	's Morgens bezoekt John zijn cliënten.

Let op!
Na werkwoorden die eindigen op een s-klank krijg je **es**.
She catches, he presses, etc.

Let op!
Na werkwoorden die eindigen op medeklinker en -y krijg je **ies** en de -y valt weg.

She cries, he flies, she applies, etc.

Grammar: the Simple Present tense

EXERCISE

Zet het woord tussen haakjes in de goede vorm.
1 He usually _____ the [diary] first. (check)
2 The GP _____ in the country. (live)
3 Every day I _____ at 8.30 am. (come in)
4 Peter always _____ a hot drink for the children. (make)
5 Jessy _____ the [elderly] people with meals. (supply)
6 He _____ free advice. (offer)
7 The child _____ her teeth every night. (brush)
8 Every night Hank _____ the practice. (clean)
9 Eve _____ her colleagues very much. (like)
10 The [welfare officer] _____ for a new job. (apply)
11 His neighbour _____ he is [fed up] with the noise. (say)
12 The [employer] _____ my cv. (check)
13 Her client _____ about a [sore] leg. (complain)
14 Every day at 1 pm all nurses _____ a cup of coffee. (have)
15 Nicky _____ in a [children's home]. (work)

1.5
Translation

Translate the following sentences.

1. Ik werk vooral met jonge mensen.

2. Zij geeft advies en uitleg.

3. Ik kom uit Nederland.

4. Ik spreek heel goed Engels.

5. Ik solliciteer naar deze functie.

1.6
Writing

Job application

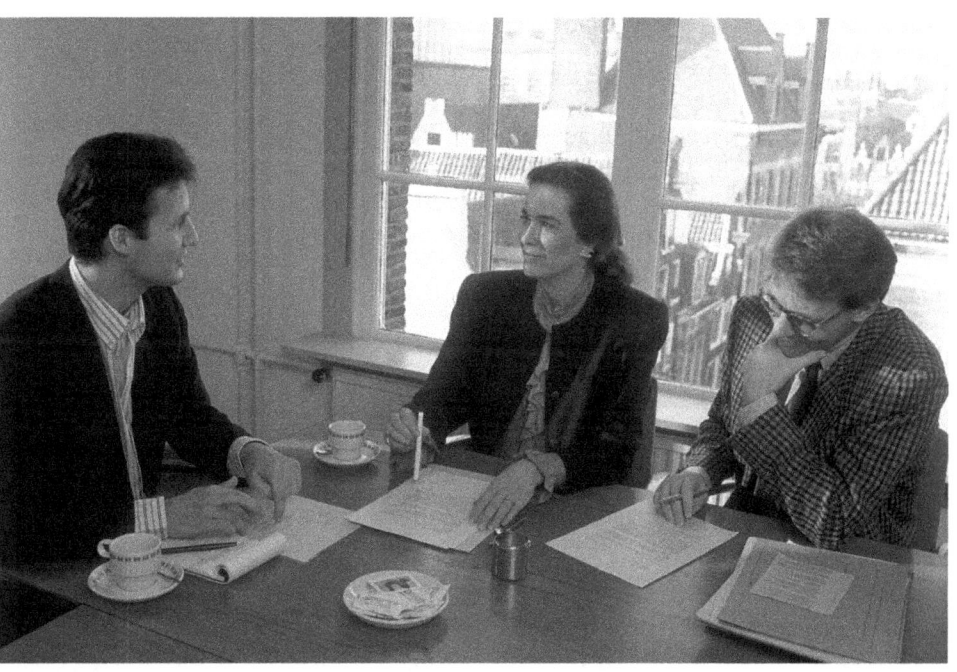

Foto: Theo Bos/Hollandse Hoogte

YOUR CV

A cv tells in short about you, your work experience and qualifications. There is no [set format], but you may find it useful to include the following:
- personal [details];
- personal profile/[career history];
- [achievements];
- work history;

- training/[qualifications];
- interests/[spare time activities];
- references.

YOUR [LETTER OF APPLICATION]

It is important that your written work makes a good first [impression]. It may be the first contact a [busy] [employer] will have with you so:
- Keep it clear and [readable].
- Do not use too many words.
- Mention your [skills] and talents clearly.
- Say something about the skills [mentioned] in the [advert].
- Be positive.
- Explain why you are perfect for the job.

Bestudeer eerst de voorbeeldbrief en schrijf dan je eigen cv en sollicitatiebrief. Kijk voor advertenties op het internet of in Engelstalige vaktijdschriften.

Name
Address
Country
Phone +31

Date

Mrs. T Black
15 North Avenue
City Health Centre
Newtown Blackshire
BLACKSHIRE BA1 5NE

Dear Mrs. Black,

I noticed your advert in the *Evening Standard* in which you offer several posts for nursing staff. I qualified as a nurse a year ago and would like to work at your Health Centre.

I have some experience working with mentally handicapped people and I would like to work in a community care setting. You will find I can work very accurately and I am very good and patient with mentally handicapped people, especially the young.

I enclose a copy of my CV. As you will see in my last job I was responsible for a team of five junior members. My last employer, Mr. Jenson, has said he will be happy to provide references for me.
I would be available to work full-time including evenings and weekends if required. I am available for an interview at your convenience and can be contacted or a message can be left at my home telephone number.

I hope to hear from you soon.

Yours sincerely,
Name XXX

1.7 Speaking

Job interview

Before you are offered a job, [usually] you will have to go for a job interview. Below are some [useful] [reminders] for a succesful interview.
At the interview:
- [Introduce] yourself.
- Be [polite] and friendly.
- Make eye contact.
- Look interested.

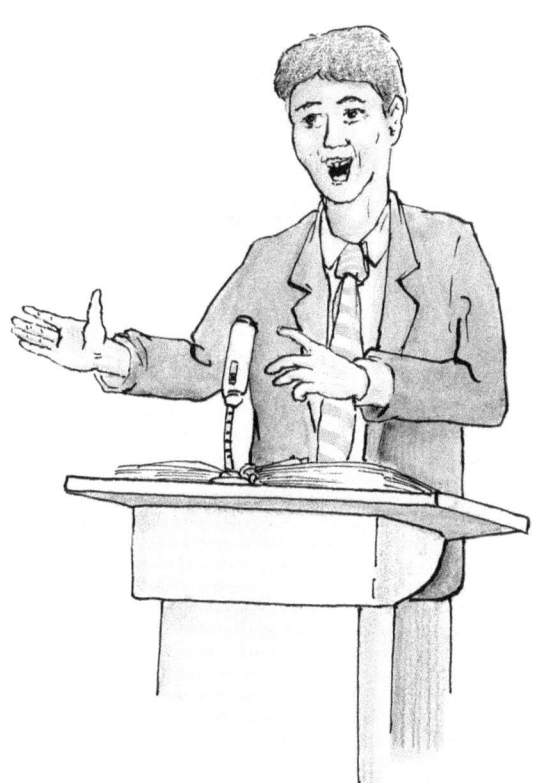

- Provide examples to [prove] your achievements.
- [Sell] yourself.
- Be positive.

Remember most employers like:
- people who listen;
- people who are [genuine];
- people who answer questions with examples;
- people who come [prepared];
- people who [appear] [confident].

Role play

Now [practice] your job interview in a role play. Work in couples. Practice the role of the [applicant] and the employer. As the employer you want to get to know your applicant by asking questions about how he or she would [deal with] for example:
- high [pressure] of work;
- [violent] [behaviour] of a client;
- [incompetent] colleagues;
- [dishonesty];
- discrimination;
- [accidents] at the workplace.

1.8
Grammar: Prepositions

Exercise

Vul een van deze voorzetsels in:
for – out – with – after – up – by – in – about – under – with – of

1. What is happening _____ this client?
2. He works _____ in the [community].
3. Keep your [records] _____ to date.
4. You look _____ the health and [welfare] of the [population].
5. What's _____ ?
6. She was _____ a lot of stress.
7. There are so many people _____ emotional or [psychological] difficulties.
8. He couldn't cope _____ his loss.
9. They work _____ [close] [partnership] with the health centre.
10. The services departments are managed _____ [local authorities].
11. To look _____ a job.
12. To work _____ a [department].
13. To look someone _____ .
14. A complaint _____ a member of staff.
15. To be employed _____ the health service.
16. I like the individual contact _____ the children and their families.
17. You will have to use a variety _____ skills.
18. The health care workers have flexibility _____ the setting they work.
19. Ask _____ a copy _____ the contract.
20. Make [arrangements] _____ people.

1.9
Research and Conversation

Networking

Most jobs are gone before they have been [advertised]. How do people know about the jobs that are [available]? That's right! Networking! Don't worry, networking isn't as difficult as it seems. In fact, most of us already [participate] in personal networking all the time. Ever asked your friends for a good [hairdresser] or [mechanic]? Well that is an example of networking.

If you want to know how to network, you should start with whom you already know. Make a list of the people that you know now or knew before and write down their job or special [skills].

People you know	Name	Job skills
[neighbours]		
(school) friends		
[colleagues]		
business [owners]		
Teachers		
Parents of your friends		
Other		

Now work in couples. After completing the list compare your information with another student.
Discuss the following items:
- Who can help you with your career?
- Which people could [benefit from] each other?
- Who you would [recommend] to someone and why?

1.10
Speaking

Presentation: improve the quality of your work

A [number] of things have gone wrong at your work. You are [in charge of] a small team.
Your boss has asked you to work out and present a [solution] for the problem. You can choose the [topic] yourself. Examples are:
- [Inappropriate] behaviour of staff
- Inappropriate behaviour of clients
- [Lack of] [safety measures]
- Nowhere to go with [complaints]
- Lack of support in the team.

Bereid een presentatie voor van ongeveer tien minuten. Vertel hierin:
- wat het probleem is;
- wat het gevolg is van het probleem;
- wat de oplossing zou kunnen zijn;
- welke rol het team hierbij heeft.
Zoek de woorden die je niet weet op in een woordenboek. Oefen de presentatie eerst in tweetallen en daarna in een grotere groep.

1.11
Grammar: the Present Continuous Tense

De *Continuous Tense* (duurvorm) wordt gevormd door **to be + het werkwoord in de -ing-vorm**.

I	*am waiting*
He/she/it	*is working*
We/you/they	*are going*

Deze vorm geeft het volgende aan:

1. Dat iets aan de gang is en kort duurt.

Are you *writing* the card?	–	Ben je de kaart aan het schrijven?
You *are working* hard today.	–	Je werkt hard vandaag.

2. Dat iets in de nabije toekomst gaat gebeuren. (Zie ook de Future Tense.)

She *is coming* to our practice tonight.	–	Ze komt vanavond naar onze praktijk.
He *is having* an operation tomorrow.	–	Morgen wordt hij geopereerd.

3. Dat iets vaak gebeurt en een negatief gevoel oproept.

Why *are* you never *helping* us?	–	Waarom help je ons nooit?
She *is* always *complaining* about pain.	–	Ze klaagt altijd over pijn.

Grammar: the Present Continuous Tense

EXERCISE

Zet het woord tussen haakjes in de goede vorm.
1 You _____ hard today. (work)
2 I _____ home now. (go)
3 She _____ for a prescription. (wait)
4 I _____ always _____ things. (lose)
5 The children _____ a lot of noise. (make)
6 It _____ heavily. (rain)
7 Tom and Mark _____ quietly. (talk)
8 The patient _____ a magazine. (read)
9 She _____ to inject herself. (learn)
10 What _____ you _____ for? (wait)

Grammar: the Simple Present Tense of the Present Continuous Tense

EXERCISE

Zet het woord tussen haakjes in de goede vorm.
1 I am tired. I _____ to bed now. (go)
2 Julie _____ German very well. (speak)
3 What time _____ the chemist's _____ (close)?
4 It _____ not _____ any more. (rain)
5 It _____ cold. (get) Shall I turn the heat up?
6 How often _____ you _____ here? (work)
7 Vegetarians _____ meat. (eat not)

8 When her husband _____ Japanese, his wife _____ English. (learn)
9 I never _____ coffee. (drink)
10 The doctor _____ at 12.30 every day. (finish)

1.12
Reading and research

Finding the right job

Choosing the right career isn't always easy. You should take the time to think about what [appeals] to you, but also [decide] which jobs [fit in] with your talents and [strengths]. When you have decided on your [career goals], do your research and find out what you need to do to get there.
The easiest thing to do is search the web for sites that offer free [career tests]. In these tests you will find questions like:

- Are you more [likely] to: act before you think?
  think before you act?
- Do you live: for what will be?
  for the moment?
- Do you trust: what you can touch?
  what you 'know'?

After you have answered all the questions you will be given a result.
Ga in tweetallen op zoek naar een Engelse website voor een beroepskeuzetest (career test).
Vul de test alle twee in en bespreek daarna of je er iets aan hebt gehad en of je het eens bent met de uitslag. Als je het niet eens bent met de uitslag zou je nog een andere test kunnen doen en daarna de uitslagen vergelijken.

2 How to survive my beliefs

2.1 Reading

Foto: Marc de Haan/
Hollandse Hoogte

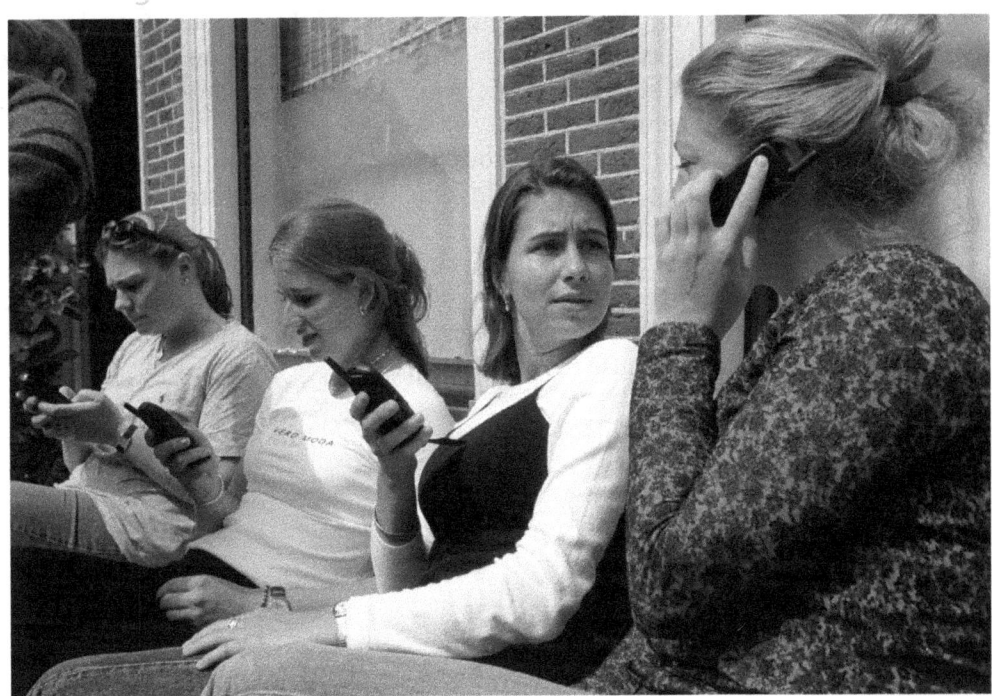

Young people need strong [voice]

The [voting age] should possibly be [lowered] to 16 as young people have 'powerful views' on many issues, [according] to [spokeswoman] Pat Thompson of children's charity Barnardo.
She presented a report to Children's Minister Margaret Hodge on Tuesday. The report does not [agree with] the idea that young people are 'politically [apathetic]'. It says many hold strong views on issues from drugs to the environment and they deserve a louder voice.
The charity took the views of more than 130 six- to 22-year-olds for its study. Pat Thompson, of Barnardo's, said the report – Give us a Chance – showed young people had 'powerful views'. She said she wanted ministers to [review] the voting age and discuss lowering it to 16.
Mrs Thompson, who is the [parliamentary adviser] with Barnardo's, said: 'All too often young people are presented as disinterested in politics, as apathetic to [decisions] and [decision making]. The young people we work with are among the most disadvantaged, yet they have powerful views that are both [considered] and [reasonable].'

The suggestions [put forward] by young people in the report include the [provision] of better [accommodation] for homeless young people, rather than [hostels]. There were also [calls for] more work in schools to [tackle] [bullying] and the view that [expulsion] is not effective in [preventing] [bad behaviour].
The youngsters who [contributed to] the report [reside] throughout the UK and covered a wide range of [subjects]. Here are some of their ideas:

'They (the [government]) say what young people should do with their lives; they should talk to the young people about what they want to do with their own lives.'
'Social services need to listen more - actually take in what the child says not [twist] it.'
'Politicians should [experience] things that affect young or [disabled] people, use a [wheelchair] or [live off] [benefits] for a week.'
'He (the [Prime Minister]) said good things about [equal opportunities]: "if you work hard you can get anywhere" is a good theory but will it really work?'
'There should be more youth groups for young people so it stops them [getting into trouble].'
'The bigger [lads] on our [estate] just hang around and make trouble, but there's nothing for them to do – the youth club's closed and you have to pay for everything else.'
'I think the government should [spend] more money on things for [teenagers] today because you get [complaints] about [vandalism] and [stuff like that] and it's because people haven't got anything better to do than be on the street, they do it because they're [bored].'

Bron: BBC news Tuesday, 18 January, 2005 and Barnardo report: Give us a Chance

Questions about the text

1. According to the text young people
a should not be allowed to vote.
b should be allowed to vote from 16.
c should be allowed to vote from 15.
d should be allowed to vote from 17.

2. *possibly* in line 1 means:
a maybe
b always
c now
d immediately

3. *report* in line 4 stands for:
a wrapped up present
b a short visit
c a campaign against child abuse
d written description of an event or situation

4. *apathetic* in line 5 means:
a showing or feeling no interest
b [ignorant]
c aggressive

d asleep

5. *environment* in line 6 refers to:
a the houses people live in
b the amount of homework
c problems with young people
d the natural world

6. *disadvantagedchildren* are children who
a are very [well off]
b have lost their parents
c are in a unfavourable situation
d argue a lot

7. According to the report young people need:
a more [pocket money].
b healthier food.
c better health care.
d better accommodation.

8. According to the report forcing someone to leave school:
a does not prevent bad behaviour.
b is not a good idea.
c can prevent bad behaviour.
d should be forbidden.

9. A *wheelchair* is a:
a chair for politicians
b chair in which you can experience life
c wheel you can sit on
d chair built on wheels for an invalid or handicapped person

10. *teenager* in line 36 refers to:
a all young people
b [adults]
c people aged between 13 and 19 years
d people aged between 8 and 12

2.2 Research

Europe on the Internet

If you look at the European site: http://europa.eu/index_en.htm you will find information that is relevant for young people. A few of the subjects [mentioned] on this site are: studying, working, [exchanges], info on Europe and [travelling] Europe.
1. Find out what the site says about working abroad. What would you have to do to work abroad?

_____

_____

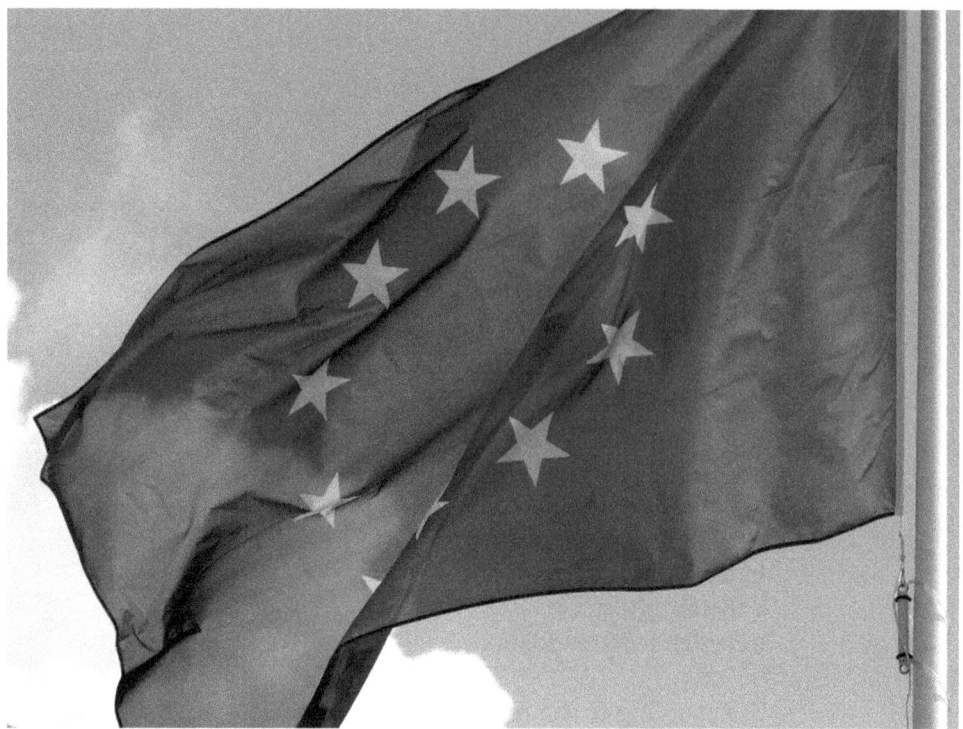

Foto: Peter Hilz/Hollandse Hoogte

2. What does it say about youth exchanges? Would you like to do that?

3. What sort of European news does it offer? Describe one news item that you find interesting or funny.

4. What portals do they have especially for young people? Which one do you like best?

5. Look for two items that you find interesting in the 'Travelling Europe' section. Describe what is in these items.

2.3
Listening Skills 2

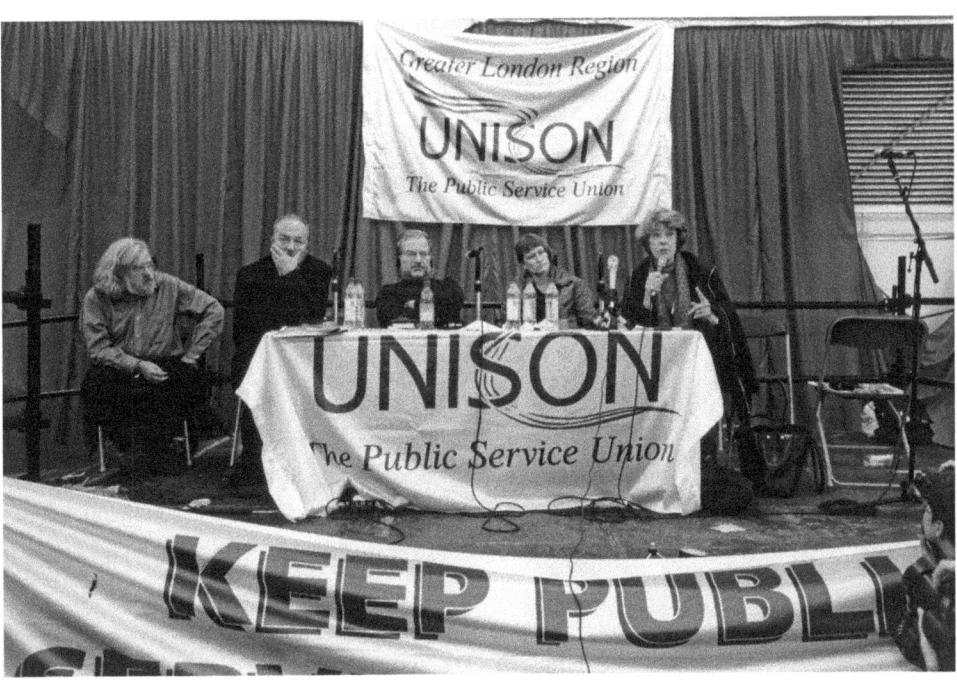

Foto: Wim Klerkx/
Hollandse Hoogte

Ten reasons for [joining] a [union]

Listen to the following conversation that took place between two [care workers] Rhona (R) and (Helen) during their [lunch break].

R: Hi Helen, how are you? You look very tired. Everything OK?

H: No, I'm bloody not OK. I'm being harassed by that [mongrel] of a boss. [Seriously] Rhona, I just don't know what to do about it. He keeps [creeping up] on me and always puts his hands on me for just a little bit too long. I told Suzie about it but she says I'm [imagining] things and that he is always like that.

R: Well, that's not an excuse, is it? Have you tried talking to him about it?

H: Oh yeah, I did that. Do you know what he did after that? He just put me on [night shift] for the rest of the week again.

R: That's terrible! He can't do that. Are you a union [member]?

H: No, I'm not. I always thought I didn't need that. Why, do you think they could help with something like this? I thought they only helped you with your contract and things like that.

R: Oh no, they can help you with all sorts of things. Here, I have a [leaflet] in my bag from Unison. It even states ten good reasons for joining. Just listen to this. [According] to them, as a union member:

- You can [earn] more.
- You're more likely to get [equal] pay.
- You get more holiday.
- You get more and better training.
- You get more [maternity leave] or [parental leave].
- You're less [likely] to be [injured] at work.
- If you do get injured at work, you'll get better compensation.
- You're less likely to be discriminated against.
- You can help keep the [public services] [public].
- You're less likely to be sacked.

H: It seems there are a lot of good reasons to join, but how can a union help me to work with my boss? It doesn't say anything about that.

R: It does actually. Just have a look at their website. If you read a bit further, then you will find all sorts of examples. I remember this story about a student nurse who was also [bullied] by her colleagues. She contacted a [workplace steward] who helped her through the entire process. I believe two people were [disciplined] and one was dismissed for his behaviour.

H: You're joking! But what if everyone [sides] with my boss? Wouldn't it be better for me to just look for another job? I don't like it that much anymore anyway.

R: You could do that, of course, but your boss will almost definitely find himself a new victim. People like that [tend to] make a habit of bullying. Someone has to stop him.

H: I'm still not [sure]. I'm so scared it is going to [turn against] me. It might just stop you know.

R You don't believe that for a minute do you? It's your call Helen. Here, take the leaflet. It says the union gives practical advice for everyone who works whether or not you're a UNISON member. [Topics] [cover] everything from your employment rights to [dealing] with stress, [handling] your boss and [juggling] work with studies. Phone them!

H: Yes, I think I will. There is nothing to lose in doing that. Thanks Rhona. I've got to go now. See you.

R Cheerio, and do call!

Idioms

Vertaal de volgende woorden uit het gesprek:

1. lastig gevallen worden –
2. vakbondslid –
3. redenen –
4. salaris –
5. schadevergoeding –
6. gediscrimineerd –
7. ontslagen –
8. voorbeelden –
9. leerling-verpleegkundige –
10. het hele stuk –
11. ontslagen –
12. gedrag –
13. grapjes maken –
14. zeker –

15. slachtoffer   –
16. gewoonte   –
17. bang   –
18. jij beslist   –
19. werknemersrechten   –
20. niets te verliezen   –

Extra questions

1. What would you do if you were Rhona?

2. What would you do if you were Helen?

3. Are you a union member? Why or why not?

2.4 Grammar: the (Simple) Past Tense (verleden tijd)

De *Simple Past Tense* wordt in de volgende gevallen gebruikt.

1. Als iets duidelijk in het verleden is gebeurd (yesterday, last week, 1992, etc.).

Last year I worked in the care for the elderly.	–	Vorig jaar werkte ik in de ouderenzorg.
Denmark joined the EU in 1973.	–	Denemarken werd in 1973 lid van de EU.

2. Als iets herhaaldelijk of volgens een schema gebeurde.

I always worked eight hours a day.	–	Ik werkte altijd acht uur per dag.
She usually went to the [child welfare office].	–	Ze ging meestal naar het bureau van de kinderbescherming.

De *Past Tense* wordt gevormd door het **hele werkwoord + ed.**

Yesterday she also **talked** to the old lady. – Gisteren sprak ze ook al met de oude vrouw.

Let op!
Bij onregelmatige werkwoorden is de verleden-tijdsvorm anders.

She broke her leg last Friday. – Afgelopen vrijdag brak ze haar been.

Bestudeer de onregelmatige werkwoorden achter in het boek (zie Appendix A).

Grammar: the Past Tense

Exercise

Kies het goede woord en zet het in de verleden tijd in onderstaande zinnen.
ask – calm – take – work – run – think – change – ring – meet – drink
1 When she was frightened, Lucy _____ her down.
2 At the end of the day she _____ away.
3 He often _____ of his mother.
4 Yesterday I _____ them for the first time
5 The child that came in this morning never _____ his clothes.
6 The man _____ me for information which I could not give him.
7 Because Mrs. Peters _____ too hard she now has high blood pressure.
8 The young father _____ the health centre almost every day.
9 He died because he _____ so much.
10 The [unruly] child _____ off.

2.5 Word Combinations

Exercise

Fill in the right verb.
1 How do you _____? (Hoe voelt u zich?)
2 How _____ you today? (Hoe gaat het vandaag met u?)
3 What do you _____? (Wat hebt u nodig?)
4 How _____ I help you? (Hoe kan ik u helpen?)
5 I _____ sick. (Ik ben misselijk.)
6 What can I _____ for you? (Wat kan ik voor u doen?)
7 He is _____ from depression. (Hij lijdt aan een depressie.)
8 Moira _____ suicide. (Moira heeft zelfmoord gepleegd.)
9 To _____ a client. (een vraaggesprek voeren met een cliënt)
10 You have to _____ for private care. (Voor particuliere zorg moet je betalen.)
11 She should _____ her GP. (Zij moet haar huisarts om raad vragen.)
12 To _____ a problem. (een probleem oplossen)
13 It will _____ no harm. (Het zal geen schade toebrengen.)
1 My boss found it hard to _____ his feelings. (Mijn baas vond het moeilijk om zijn gevoelens te tonen.)
2 Anyone who _____ help may apply. (Iedereen die hulp nodig heeft, kan een verzoek indienen.)

2.6 Speaking

Role play: I Want change

When you are not happy about, for example, the amount of homework you have to do or the way your teachers treat you, you can try and change this. You could do this by

3. Do you think it is a good idea to have students represent other students? Why (not)?

2.8 Translation

Exercise

Translate the following sentences.

1. Ze protesteerde tegen zijn slechte gedrag.

2. Greenpeace is een heel bekende belangengroep.

3. Zij kozen drie studenten.

4. De studenten besloten te gaan stemmen.

5. Hij verbeterde de kwaliteit van de school.

2.9 Write your own campaign or party programme

Schrijf je eigen campagne of partijprogramma. Werk in tweetallen.
Think of a subject or political party you feel very strongly about. In the campaign or party programme the following should be clear:
- the reason for the campaign or programme;
- what the campaign or party programme is all about;
- who the campaign or party programme is aimed at;
- what you hope to [achieve] with the campaign or party programme.

Examples of subjects could be:
- animal welfare;

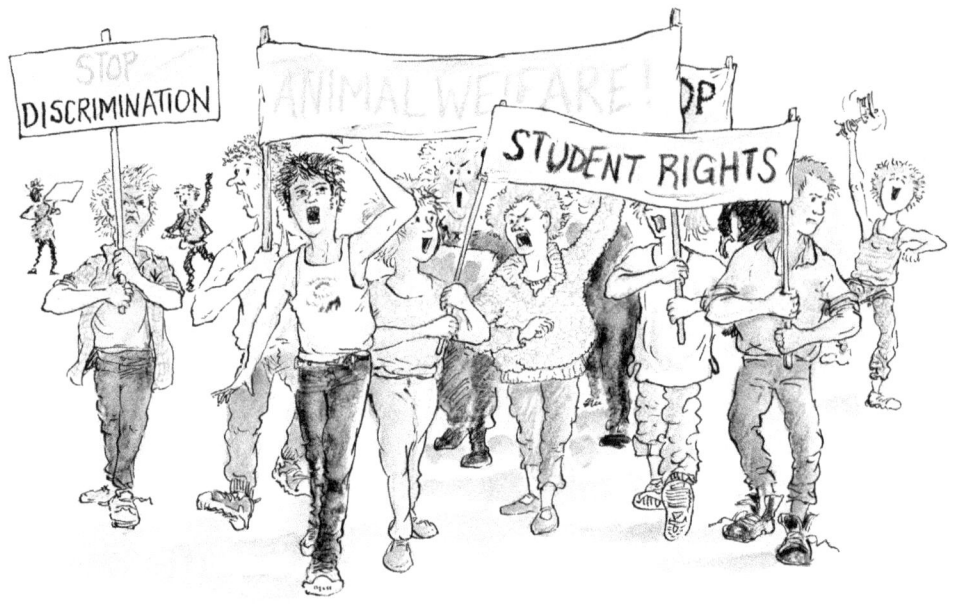

- students rights;
- equality;
- freedom of culture;
- freedom of education;
- safe sex;
- discrimination;
- free housing.

But you can also think of a subject yourself!

2.10
Reading

Read the following views on Europe.

A Window on Europe: what do you think?

Katy Gilmour, 16, from Dunblane, still in school
'I think that the Euro is [probably] inevitable. At the moment, I think we should be more involved in Europe, otherwise we will just get more isolated. I don't think we hear enough about the European Parliament: I have a [vague] knowledge of the people that represent me in Europe. I have no idea when the next European elections are.'

Hannah MacKenzie, 16, from Milngavie, still in school
'I'm not that interested in politics. It doesn't really [affect] me, as I'm too young to vote. Sometimes politicians don't listen to young people. They should have a kind of committee of children to speak to the government.
I think the Euro is a good thing, and it seems to be working everywhere else. I'm not sure what the European Parliament does, but it seems like a good idea. I

would always say I'm Scottish, never British. I think that's because the rest of Britain is quite different, in terms of [laws].'

David Stevenson, 17, from Glasgow
'I've just come back from Barcelona and the thing that really [struck] me was how much more healthily people eat. Walking through the streets, you notice far fewer [obese] people. Otherwise, I don't think we are very different from the rest of Europe.
I'm not really aware of the European Parliament and what it does compared to the Scottish Parliament and Westminster.
Young people are not really represented in politics, but then there are a lot of people my age who have unreasonable views, so maybe it is a bit [unwise] to give people my age that responsibility.'

Jonny Mowlem, 17, is a [sales assistant] from Edinburgh
'Europe's very diverse. I'm quite glad that no European countries are like America and Iraq are just now. If you were to ask if I was European or British, I'd probably say British. But if I was maybe 10 years older and I'd been on holiday a couple more times, maybe I'd say more European.
I think that the currency we have is strong. I don't think it should change. Scotland's place in Europe is small, but we've got a good image abroad.'

Bron: The Herald June 27, 2006 Copyright © 2006 Newsquest (Herald & Times) Limited

Idioms

Find the following words in the text above.

1. onvermijdelijk   -
2. stemmen   -
3. betrokken   -
4. anders   -
5. het lijkt   -
6. kennis   -
7. regering   -
8. vertegenwoordigen   -
9. gezonder   -
10. verantwoordelijkheid   -
11. commissie   -
12. vekiezingen   -
13. uiteenlopend   -
14. europees parlement   -
15. vergeleken met   -
16. waarschijnlijk   -
17. buitenland   -
18. onredelijke meningen   -

19. munt, geldstelsel –
20. wetten –

Extra questions

1. What do you think about Europe?

2. Do you agree with anyone in the text? Why (not)?

3. Do you think all European countries should use the Euro? Why (not)?

2.11
Speaking

Lees eerst in de voorbeelden welk advies er bij een aantal problemen wordt gegeven.

What to do if people don't treat you right?

Example 1
How can I deal with stress at work?
The best thing you can do with stress is to know how to:
- [recognise] it;
- [avoid] it when possible;
- [handle] it where [necessary];
- get support when you need it from friends, colleagues;
- know when stress is a serious problem and you need [union] or specialist advice.

Learn to:
- respect yourself;
- know your [limits];
- say no to [unreasonable] [demands];

- ask others for help;
- set realistic [goals];
- not [overdo] it;
- manage your time well;
- take one day at a time;
- keep it in [perspective];
- stop [critisizing] yourself;
- relax;
- [treat] yourself.

[Destressing]:
There are lots of different ways to destress which involve looking after yourself and learning how to relax no matter how bad a day you're having. Different techniques [suit] different people so try things out to find out what works for you. Here's a few ideas:
- [controlled deep breathing] and meditation;
- [visualisation];
- massage – it doesn't have to cost money just ask a friend;
- [physical exercise] and fresh air;
- walk to work, cycle, swim in your lunch break;
- [stretching] in the office to reduce [muscle tension] and prevent [strain];
- take [breaks] at work, eat [regularly], healthy food;
- do not use too much caffeine, alcohol, salt and sugar;
- do something for yourself that you enjoy every day - make time for a hot bath, a TV soap, read a book.

Example 2
I think I'm being [bullied] at work – what can I do?
The first thing is to be clear about what is unacceptable, [bullying] [behaviour]. Bullying includes:
- [violence] or the [threat] of violence;
- [calling you names] or making jokes about you;
- constant criticism;
- shouting at you;
- [humiliating] you or [picking on] you in front of others or in private;
- making you [fail] by, for example, [overloading] you with work;
- always making you do the worst or most difficult tasks;
- [general] [rudeness] and [unpleasantness];
- spreading [lies and rumours] about you.

You can be bullied by anyone, whether it's your boss, a [co-worker] or a [customer]. Some kinds of bullying are more [obvious] than others. The bullying can happen anytime, anyplace, anywhere. Don't [put up with] being bullied. It's [unfair] and bad for your health.
Your first [aim] is for the bullying to stop. You may also want the bully to be [disciplined].
- Tell the bully to stop.
- If there are other [witnesses] ask them to [note down] what they saw or heard.
- Tell someone else [immediately] – a friend, colleague or someone [senior].
- Keep a [diary] of [each] [incident] large and small – date, time, place.

- Write to the bully following any incidents, [denying] or [correcting] their [false claims] if necessary. - [Keep] copies of any [correspondence] as [evidence].

Employers do have a general [legal duty] to [protect] the health and [safety] of [employees]. Bullying may be sexual or racial which may mean it is also [unlawful] discrimination.
People who bully should be disciplined or in the worst cases [dismissed] for their behaviour.

Bron: Unison 2006

Werk in tweetallen. Bedenk samen een voorbeeld van een probleem of ongepast gedrag dat zou kunnen voorkomen bij jou op de werkvloer. Beschrijf de situatie eerst op papier. Speel daarna een rollenspel waarbij één student een vertrouwenspersoon speelt en de ander iemand die van iets of iemand last heeft en hierover wil vertellen. In het gesprek moet aan de orde komen:
— *wat het probleem is;*
— *hoe lang het al speelt;*
— *waarom je er last van hebt;*
— *wat je er zelf aan gedaan hebt om het op te lossen;*
— *wat je van de vertrouwenspersoon verwacht;*
— *hoe je ervoor kunt zorgen dat het in de toekomst niet weer gebeurt.*

3 How to survive my organization

3.1 Reading

Foto: Bert Beelen/
Hollandse Hoogte

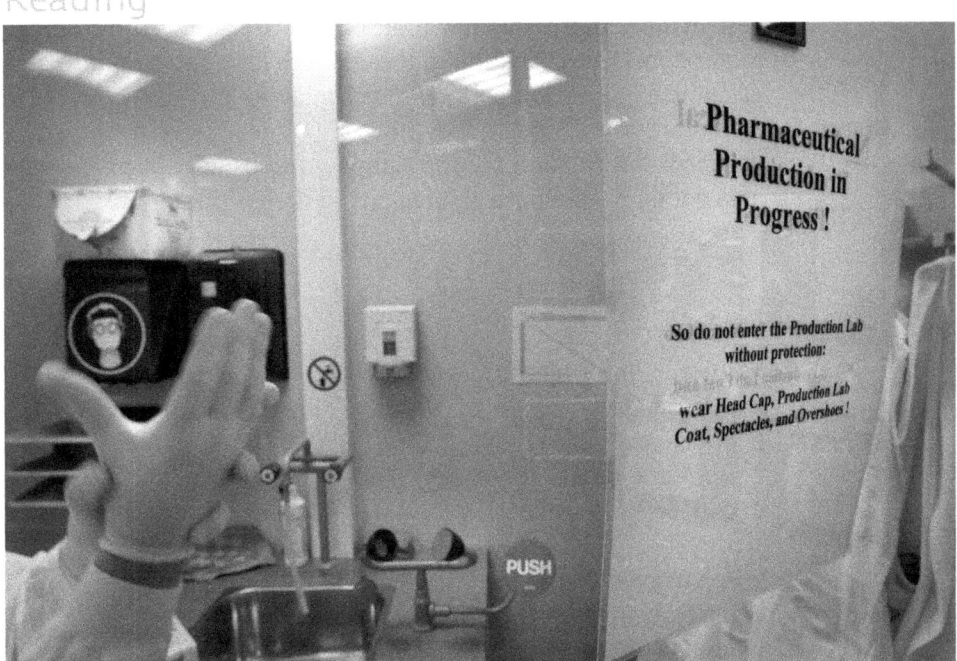

Read the following text.

Too many young people are getting [hurt] at work

Across Europe, 18 to 24-year-olds are at least 50% more [likely] to be [injured] in the workplace than more [experienced] workers. Behind the [statistics] are harrowing stories, of young people having to live with the consequences of accidents and [damaged] health for the rest of their lives, or dying when they had so much of their lives ahead of them.
Employers need to do more to protect young workers, and young people need to be more aware of health and [safety issues] when they enter the world of work.
That is why the Safe Start [campaign] is being [launched]. Safe Start is [dedicated] to [improving] the [occupational safety] and health (OSH) of the EU's 75 million young people.
[Announcing] the [launch], EU [Commissioner] for [Employment], [Social Affairs] and [Equal Opportunities] said that young workers' safety wasn't just a [matter] for young people themselves: 'Our message is that we all share responsibility for [protecting] young people at work. Employers have a [duty of care] and are [legally] responsible for the health and safety of their workers. EU law [recognises] that young

people need special [protection]. But this is also an issue for parents, for health and safety professionals, and for the education community. And [ultimately], it's an issue for [policymakers]. We all have to work together, to make sure that young people have a safe and healthy start to their working lives.'

As well as making employers and young workers more aware of risks, Safe Start aims to [involve] educators in an important role. As the Director of the European Agency for Safety and Health at Work, [explains]: 'We can't just leave it until young people have already started work to teach them about health and safety. We have to reach them early on – while they are still at school or college – so that they get used to a culture of risk prevention.'

'With the world of work changing so quickly, this deep-rooted "health and safety thinking" will help young people deal with whatever risks they may [face] throughout their working lives. It should be [part and parcel] of the school and college curriculum. We also want our engineers, designers, architects, medical students and business managers of tomorrow to be risk-aware and well-informed about OSH in their professional roles. [Instilling] these values in young people at an early age will help to promote a prevention culture in workplaces.'

For more information see the campaign website at http://ew2006.osha.eu.int and help young people have a Safe Start to their working lives.

Questions about the text

1. *across* in line 1 means:
a opposed to
b opposite
c from one side to the other
d outside

2. A harrowing story is a:
a distressing story.
b funny story.
c sad story.
d [boring] story.

3. *consequence* in line 3 means:
a pain
b thought
c idea
d a result or effect

4. *To be aware* means:
a to know about.
b to forget about.
c to think about.
d to warn about.

5. OSH refers to:
a [first aid].
b occupational [hazard].
c occupational health.
d occupational safety and health.

6. *To share responsibility* means:
a one person is responsible.
b more people are responsible.
c no one is responsible.
d the EU is responsible.

7. Safe Start wants to:
a include educators.
b exclude educators.
c be a role model for educators.
d warn educators.

8. *Deep-rooted* means:
a thoughtful.
b long roots.
c firmly placed.
d deep thoughts.

9. *a curriculum* in line 28 refers to:
a the details of an applicant
b a university course
c all the subjects tou like
d the subjects of a course or study

10. *values* in line 31 refers to:
a standards of behaviour
b how much something is worth
c how much you earn
d how valuable you are

3.2
Listening Skill 4

Performance interview

Souraya (S) has been working in Holy Corner Health Center for three months. After her probation she has a [performance interview] with her boss Gita (G).

G: Sit down Souraya, can I get you coffee or tea?

S: Thank you, [white coffee] please.

G: We will have a look at your performance [sheets] in a minute. First, I would like to know how you feel about your job thus far.

S: Erm... well, what I think? I think it is a very nice job although it is very demanding and I think I still have to learn a lot of things.

G: When you say demanding what do you mean, what do you find most difficult?

S: I think the gravity of the problems that people have and the way they don't take responsibility for the mess they are in... that's what I find hard.

G: What efforts have you made to improve yourself in this?

S: I ask the others about it and I have started reading up on things but I don't know if that is enough.

G: Well it always helps to be better informed. Do you feel insecure when you work with clients?

S: I do sometimes, especially when they know so much more about their condition than I do.

G: What do you do when that happens?

S: Well, I sometimes go to the office and look things up. If can't find any information I ask one of my colleagues.

G: Does the client not have to wait for a very long time then?

S: Erm... Yea... erm I don't know what else to do in a situation like that. When clients phone you can always call them back but when they come in for an appointment...

G: Well that's why it is so important to ask why somebody wants to come in. So you can prepare yourself and have all the details you need.

S: I suppose so.

G: Don't look like that. You have nothing to worry about, look at these reports. Most of them say: Fully Achieves Expectations. There is only one that says: Needs improvement to fully achieve expectations. But who doesn't need improvement?

S: Well, I certainly do.

G: You have only been here three months Souraya. You will get the hang of it in no time. Just trust yourself to do the right thing. Do you have any other issues or concerns that we can work on together?

S: Erm... I don't think so, for now.

G: Well, off you go then, enjoy your day.

S: Thank you, bye.

Idioms

Vertaal de volgende woorden uit het gesprek:

1. Proeftijd –
2. Tot nu toe –
3. Veeleisend –
4. Ernst –
5. Verantwoordelijkheid –
6. Puinhoop –
7. Pogingen –
8. verbeteren –
9. Onzeker –
10. Aandoening –
11. Afspraak –
12. Voorbereiden –
13. Rapporten –
14. Bereikt –
15. verwachtingen –
16. verbetering –
17. Onder de knie krijgen –
18. Problemen –
19. genieten –

3.3
Conversation

When things go wrong

First read the two [case studies].

[ELDER] [ABUSE] CASE STUDY

The Professional [Conduct Committee] examined the case of a [registered] [mental health nurse], (RMN). The nurse [faced] seven [allegations] made [whilst] he worked over a period of nearly nine months as a mental health nurse at the [nursing unit] of a [nursing home].
The [circumstances] of the case:
The charges against the nurse [included] [restraining] a patient by standing on his foot. The patient [concerned] was in his eighties and [suffered from] dementia. After the patient had become upset and [agitated] the nurse put his foot down the patient's [shin] to rest on his foot to restrain him. The nurse was stopped by a [care assistant] who pushed him away after seeing the [incident].
The second charge involved restraining another patient, in his sixties, also suffering from dementia, on the floor in an [inappropriate] manner. After a fight between two [residents] the nurse [pinned] one patient to the ground by sitting on top of him after he had fallen.
The nurse was also charged with [responding] to a [care assistant's] [request] for a patient's [bandages] to be [changed], with words similar to, 'She can bleed. I'm [fed up] of changing them'. The patient concerned suffered from a [skin condition] that meant her bandages often needed changing. [Although] the nurse had changed the bandages more than once earlier that day he refused when the care assistant requested his help.

Social worker [removed] from register after [misconduct] found

The [independent] [Conduct Committee] of the General Social Care Council [GSCC] yesterday decided the case of a social worker from Halesowen who was alleged to have [breached] the codes of practice by having an inappropriate relationship with a [service user].
Misconduct was found against John Anthony, and he was removed from the Social Care Register.
Social workers work with people who are often [vulnerable]. It is unacceptable for a social worker to abuse the [trust] placed in them by discriminating against an individual, putting them at [unnecessary] risk or forming an inappropriate personal relationship. The GSCC [exists] to promote high standards [among] social care workers and can take action against those who do not [meet] the standards [laid down] in the codes of practice. At the same time, we [applaud] the many thousands of social care workers who meet those standards and do so much to help the people in their care.

Werk in groepjes van vier. Voer een discussie over wanneer iemand uit het register moet worden verwijderd. Eerst bedenk je samen over welk wangedrag je het gaat hebben. Eén persoon is voor verwijdering uit het register en minstens één persoon is tegen. Eén persoon is discussieleider (zie onderstaande tips). De discussieleider zorgt ervoor dat iedereen evenveel aan het woord komt en dat er naar elkaar geluisterd wordt. Aan het einde van de discussie geeft de discussieleider een samen-

vatting van wat er gezegd is. Eventueel nabespreken met de hele groep of wisselen van rol of onderwerp. Hieronder staan enkele voorbeeldzinnen die je zou kunnen gebruiken.

Tips voor de discussieleider

Denk aan de volgende zaken:
- Be an active listener.
- [Repeat] information.
- Use [body language].
- [Refer] to [participants] by name.
- Use [kind] words.
- Speak [clearly].
- Don't dominate the discussion.
- Help participants who are [looking for] words.
- [Cut off] dominant speakers [gently] by saying: 'That was interesting, now let's hear others.'

Helpful phrases to use in the discussion

Beginnen met de discussie:

First of all / For a start	–	Ten eerste
To begin with	–	Om mee te beginnen
I'd start by	–	Ik zou willen beginnen met
There're two points here: firstly... secondly...	–	Er zijn twee punten hier ten eerste... ten tweede...

Mening geven:

In my opinion / In my view	–	Naar mijn mening
I strongly believe in	–	Ik ben ervan overtuigd dat
I definitely think that	–	Ik denk zeker dat
Don't you think it's better to	–	Denk je niet dat het beter is om
I'd agree with you if	–	Ik ben het met je eens als
But surely	–	Het is toch zeker zo
Yes, but	–	Ja, maar
That may be so, but	–	Dat is misschien zo maar
I agree.	–	Ik ben het ermee eens.
I disagree entirely.	–	Ik ben het er helemaal niet mee eens.
I'm afraid I can't agree.	–	Ik ben bang dat ik het er niet mee eens ben.

Om meer informatie vragen:

Can you be a bit more specific?	–	Kun je er wat meer over zeggen?
Does that happen?	–	Gebeurt dat?
What do you mean?	–	Wat bedoel je?
In what way?	–	Hoe bedoel je?
Why do you say that?	–	Waarom zeg je dat?
Why's that?	–	Waarom is dat?
Are we talking about	–	Hebben we het over
Are you saying that	–	Wil je zeggen dat
What are you trying to say?	–	Wat wil je zeggen?

Meer informatie geven:

Let me explain.	–	Laat me het uitleggen.
I'm saying that / I mean.	–	Ik bedoel
I think	–	Ik denk
To my experience	–	In mijn ervaring

3.4 Grammar: the Future Tense (toekomende tijd)

De *Future Tense* wordt in de volgende situatie gebruikt.

1. Als iets op een bepaald of onbepaald moment in de toekomst gebeurt.

The doctor will see her patient tomorrow.	–	De dokter gaat morgen bij haar patiënt langs.
This afternoon she is going to the shops.	–	Vanmiddag gaat ze naar de winkels.

De *Future Tense* wordt gevormd door **shall** of **will + hele werkwoord**.
Shall gebruik je alleen bij *I* en *we*. **Will** mag je altijd gebruiken.
Voor de nabije toekomst mag je ook gebruiken **BE + going to**.

I *shall explain* to you what you must do.	–	Ik zal u uitleggen wat u moet doen.
We *will read* the brochure.	–	We zullen de brochure lezen.
Susan *is going to* speak with her client.	–	Susan gaat met haar cliënt praten.

Zowel **shall** als **will** mag je afkorten tot **'ll**.

I'll eat healthier food from now on.	–	Vanaf nu zal ik gezonder eten.

Grammar: the Future Tense

EXERCISE

Geef aan of onderstaande zinnen goed of fout zijn en verbeter de foute zinnen.

1. I shall have a look on the internet to find out more about this organization.

2. Mike shall help that client when he has finished this [chore].

3. Next week Hassan goes to the [refugee centre].

4. I hope the next [counsellor] is going to be a bit friendlier.

5. The new [stock] arrives at 4 pm.

6. From now on I am working harder to get the work done on time.

7. Shall we go together to the [Health Education] Class this evening?

8. If you eat enough vitamins you shall feel much better.

9. My colleague will walk you to the [exit].

10. Anne said she is making coffee this afternoon.

3.5 Translation

Exercise

Translate the following sentences:

1. Wees niet bang om vragen te stellen.

2. Je moet al je medicijnen bij dezelfde apotheek halen.

3. Als u het moeilijk vindt om te onthouden, moet u het opschrijven.

4. Hier is een folder met wat informatie.

5. Over deze apparaten hebben we informatie beschikbaar.

3.6 Listening Skills 5

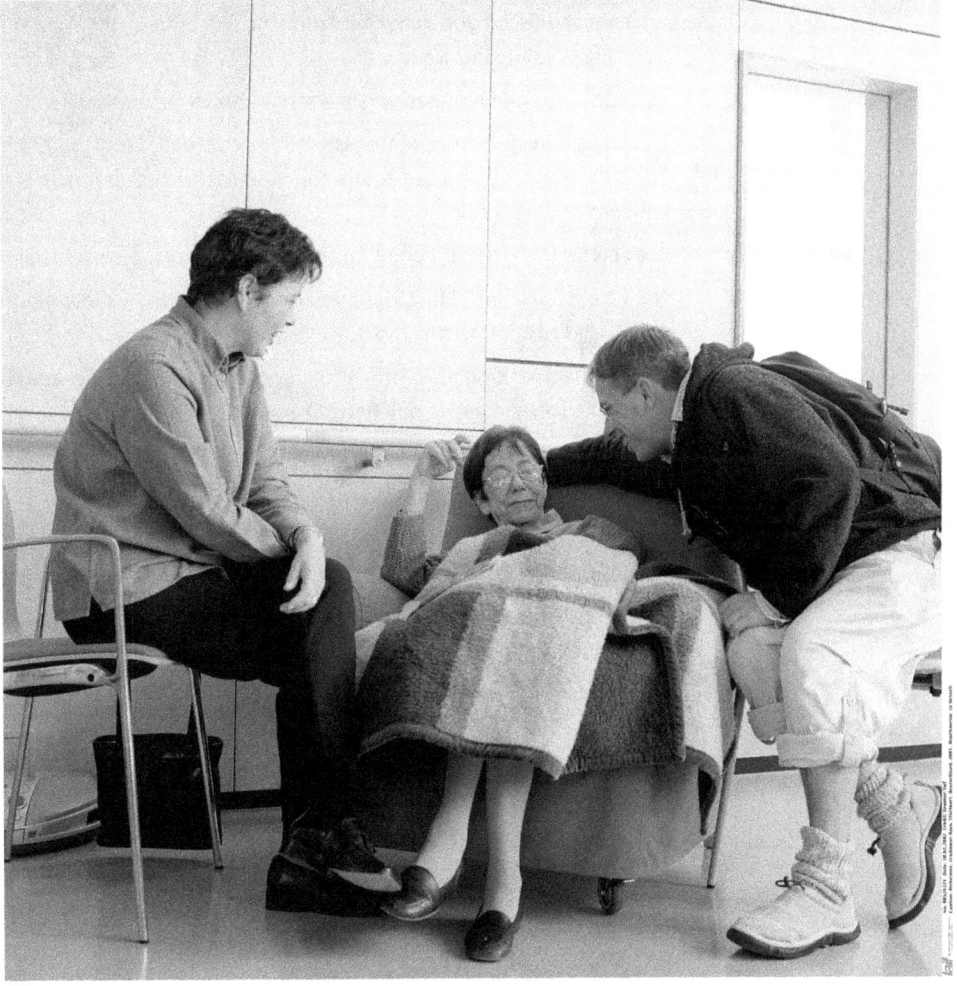

Foto: Lait/Hollandse Hoogte

Can you help us?

Mr. Ashar is suffering from Alzheimer's disease. After he [deteriorated] he was taken to hospital. The hospital staff feels he has to be [transferred] to a nursing home. A social care worker (S) and a nurse (N) discuss the transfer with Mr. Ashar's wife Amrita (A) and daughter Sadvhi (D).

S: Good morning Mrs. Ashar and Miss Ashar. We are here to discuss Mr. Ashar's situation. The staff here feels he is not well enough to go back home. They have asked me if he would be [eligible] for a place in a nursing home. How would you feel about that?

A: No madam, I would like to take my husband home, thank you.

S: I understand you want to keep your husband close to you Mrs. Ashar, but he needs so much specialist care and attention. We feel it might even be dangerous if he remains at home. He will keep [wandering off].

A: My daughter and I can look after him. We have always done so.

N: But your daughter needs to have her own life too, what about her education or work?

A: She has never complained about it. That is how we do things you know. We look after each other as a family. Don't we Sadvhi?

D: Mm...

N: How do you feel about all this Sadvhi? Do you want your father to come home too?

D: Er. It's very difficult you know. I do think he will be very unhappy in a nursing home, but I don't know how long we can...

A: Of course he will be unhappy. He doesn't know those people.

N: But what if he gets hurt again? This time your [neighbour] found him in time, but he could have burnt the house down. You have to think of your own [safety] and that of your children as well you know.

A: Are you saying I'm not a good mother? That I don't look after them [properly]?

N: No, no of course not. I just want you [to look ahead]. In a few months time you won't be able to look after him any more.

S: You can help looking after him in the nursing home too, if that's what you want. Why don't you go and have a look first? See what it is all about?

D: Maybe we should Mum. We can always [decide] after that.

S: Would you like me to come along?

A: No thank you, we can have a look for ourselves. I knew I should not have brought him to hospital. He told me: 'they will never let me go again.' He was right you know.

N: But we are only trying to help. Alzheimer is a serious disease. There is a lot of [expertise] in the nursing home. There are special [wards] with people with the same [condition]. All the staff have been [trained] to deal with the problems you are dealing with all alone now.

A: I have never complained!

S: I will make an [appointment] for your visit and we will discuss it again after that. Can you agree to that?

D: Yes, we will go and have a look, won't we Mum?

A: But I won't agree to anything yet. As long as that is clear. (*stands up and leaves*)

S: You won't have to, first just go and have a look. See what you think. You can always call me if you have any questions. Bye for now.

Exercise

Geef aan of de volgende beweringen juist (true) of onjuist (false) zijn.

1. After Mr. Ashar became worse he was taken to hospital. *true / false*
2. The GP feels Mr. Ashar has to be transferred to a nursing home. *true / false*
3. Mrs. Ashar wants to take her husband home. *true / false*
4. The daughter thinks it is dangerous if her dad [remains] at home. *true / false*
5. The hospital staff is afraid Mr. Ashar will keep walking away. *true / false*
6. Sadvhi has never complained about looking after her dad. *true / false*
7. Sadvhi thinks Mr. Ashar will be happy in a nursing home. *true / false*
8. The hospital has special wards with people with Alzheimer's disease. *true / false*
9. The social care worker makes an appointment for a visit to the nursing home. *true / false*
10. In the end Mrs. Ashar agrees to the transfer. *true / false*

3.7 Fluency: How to give advice

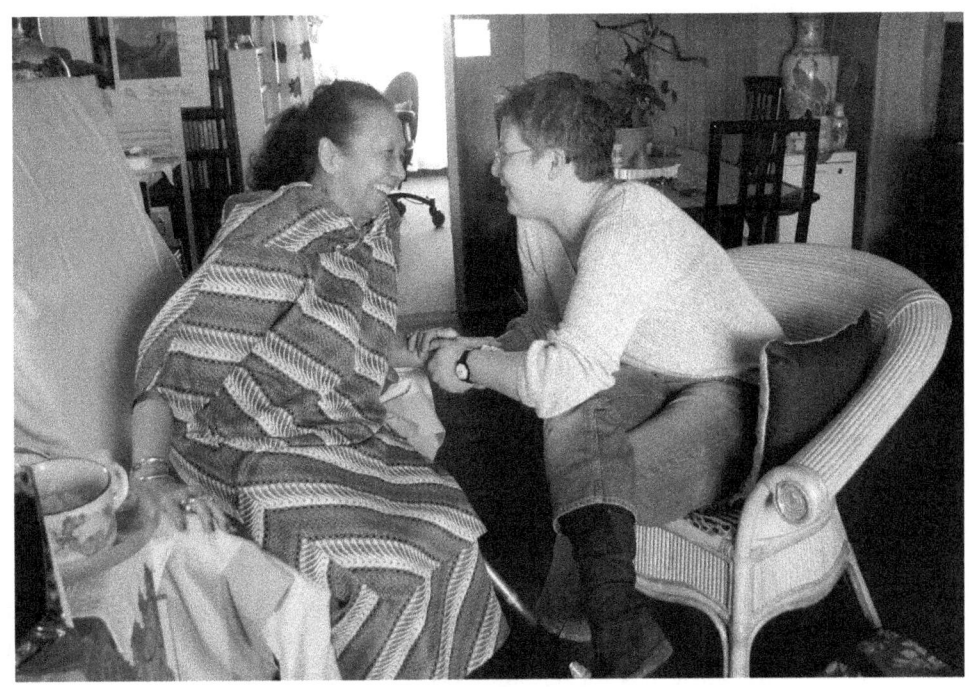

Foto: Bert Spiertz/ Hollandse Hoogte

When you give advice make sure:
– you tune (afstemmen op) your advice to your patient's/client's need (*behoefte*);

- you know how well your patient/client can process (verwerken) the information;
- you are familiar with (bekend met) your patient's/client's social environment (sociale omgeving);
- you are familiar with your patient's/client's living and working situation;
- you are informed of the advice and treatment given so far (tot nu toe).

Phrases that can be used by nursing staff / social care workers:
- What is the problem?
- How long have you been suffering from this problem?
- Does it hurt (pijn)?
- When does it hurt?
- What sort of treatment have you tried before?
- Do you have any other complaints (klachten)?
- What have you done to solve the problem thus far?
- Who can help you at home?
- How do you feel about the things that have happened?
- Why do you think this has happened?
- Is there anyone in your family with the same problem?

Phrases that can be used by patients/clients
- I don't feel very well.
- I have been ill since...
- I have a terrible (ontzettende) pain in...
- My child doesn't want to...
- I have been suffering from...
- I can't use my...
- My medication doesn't work/is out of date (verlopen)/is finished...
- I don't know how to...
- I have large debts (schulden)
- I have a problem with alcohol/drugs/gambling (gokken)
- I can't cope with...
- I feel depressed/sad/angry about...
- I don't know how to...

Exercise

Now find a partner and practice a conversation between a nurse or social care worker and a patient/client in different situations. You can make one up or choose one of the following situations:

1. A nurse is asked by a male patient who has just found out he has an STD (Sexual Transmitted Disease: seksueel overdraagbare aandoening) whether he should tell his girlfriend.
Words you can use are: responsibility, honesty, precautions, condom, multiple sexual contacts (verantwoordelijkheid, eerlijkheid, voorzorgsmaatregelen, condoom, wisselende contacten).

2. A social care worker receives a phone call from a mother. She has just found out her fifteen-year-old daughter has been using heroin and stealing to get enough money to pay for her addiction.
Words you can use are: underage, detoxification programme, drug rehabilitation centre, self-help group, support groups (minderjarig, afkickbehandeling, afkickcentrum, zelfhulpgroep, steungroepen).

3.8
Grammar: Much, many, little, few

Much (veel) en **little** (weinig) worden gebruikt voorafgaand aan ontelbare zelfstandige naamwoorden (zelfstandige naamwoorden die je níet kunt tellen).

much time	–	veel tijd
much luck	–	veel geluk
little energy	–	weinig energie
little money	–	weinig geld

Many (veel) en **few** (weinig) worden gebruikt voor telbare zelfstandige naamwoorden (zelfstandige naamwoorden die je wél kunt tellen).

many friends	–	veel vrienden
many people	–	veel mensen
few pills	–	weinig pillen
few infants	–	weinig zuigelingen

Exercise

Zet het woord tussen haakjes in de goede vorm.
1 I did not spend _____ money. (veel)
2 How _____ people are there still in the waiting room? (veel)
3 He has very _____ pills left. (weinig)
4 I do not go out _____ . (veel)
5 There is _____ time. (weinig)

3.9
Writing

Happy at work

How happy you are at work [depends] on yourself, your colleagues, your boss, your [salary] and where you work. Find out what you would like in your job to make you happy. Make a top 5 of the five best and worst things a job can offer. When you are finished, compare your top 5 with a fellow student. Discuss the [differences] and [similarities].

The best thing about my job is	The worst thing about my job is
1.	1.
2.	2.
3.	3.
4.	4.
5.	5.

3.11
Grammar: a or an

In het Engels wordt een zelfstandig naamwoord dat met een klinker begint voorafgegaan door **an**, bijvoorbeeld *an assistant*. Een zelfstandig naamwoord dat met een medeklinker begint wordt voorafgegaan door **a**, bijvoorbeeld: *a client*.
Deze regel heeft echter betrekking op de uitspraak van het woord en níet op de schrijfwijze. Om die reden is het: **an** *hour* en níet *a hour*.

Exercise

Vul in: **a** or **an**.

CHILDLINE STORIES

Jake, 1) _____ 16-year old boy, called ChildLine because he was worried about his mum. 'I can't sleep at night. I stay awake until my mum goes to sleep. I'm afraid she'll kill herself.'
Jake said his mum had tried to kill herself 2) _____ number of times. She once slit her wrists. This happened mostly after his parents argued or she had 'one of her attacks'.
He said, 'They can be fine for 3) _____ hour or so but then they start to argue again and sometimes they scream that it was 4) _____ mistake for them to have me and my little brother. And they say personal things about each other that we don't like to hear. The shouting scares my brother and I have to look after him.' 5) _____ older sister left the house years ago.
Jake said when his mum threatened to kill herself, his dad acted like he didn't care and it was Jake who had to try to stop her and calm her down. This made him angry with his dad.
Jake wanted to tell his parents how he felt, but was afraid that if he did, his mum might try to kill herself again, or that his dad might throw him out. He said he felt very alone, with no support. The ChildLine counsellor suggested that if Jake found it hard to talk to his parents, he should write them 6) _____ note, telling them how he felt.
A week later, Jake called again. He had written a note to his parents telling them how their rows and his mum's suicide attempts made him and his brother feel. His parents were really shocked and said they didn't realise how bad it had been for Jake and his brother.

3.12
Conversation

Coaching

Sinds kort moet jij je jongere collega's begeleiden en evalueren. Dit gaat meestal goed maar soms ook niet. In deze oefening ga je een evaluatiegesprek naspelen met een collega die zich niet aan de regels of afspraken houdt. Je mag een van de situaties nemen die hier worden genoemd of zelf een situatie verzinnen.

During the [evaluation] you:
– state the problems;

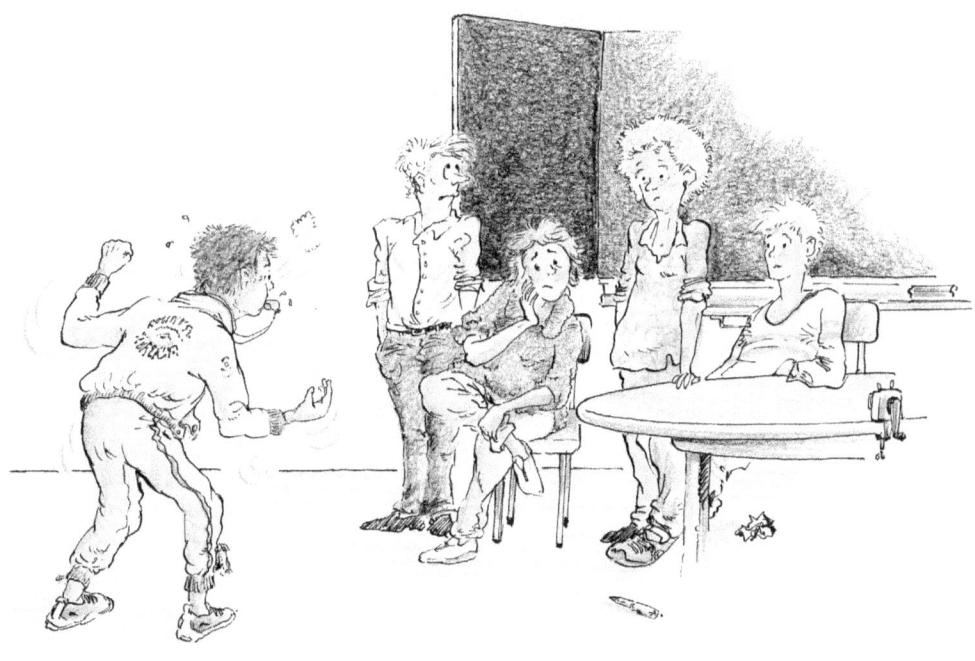

- state negative and positive points;
- remain respectful and understanding;
- explain why something is wrong;
- look for solutions to solve the problem ;
- tell your colleague when the next meeting will be.

Situations you can use are:
- your colleague is always late;
- your colleague is not very respectful towards clients;
- your colleague discriminates;
- your colleague is not always honest;
- your colleague does not work very hard;
- your colleague is not a teamworker;
- your colleague abuses her power.

4 How to survive my shopping?

4.1 How to choose a mobile service

Foto: Rien Zilvold/
Hollandse Hoogte

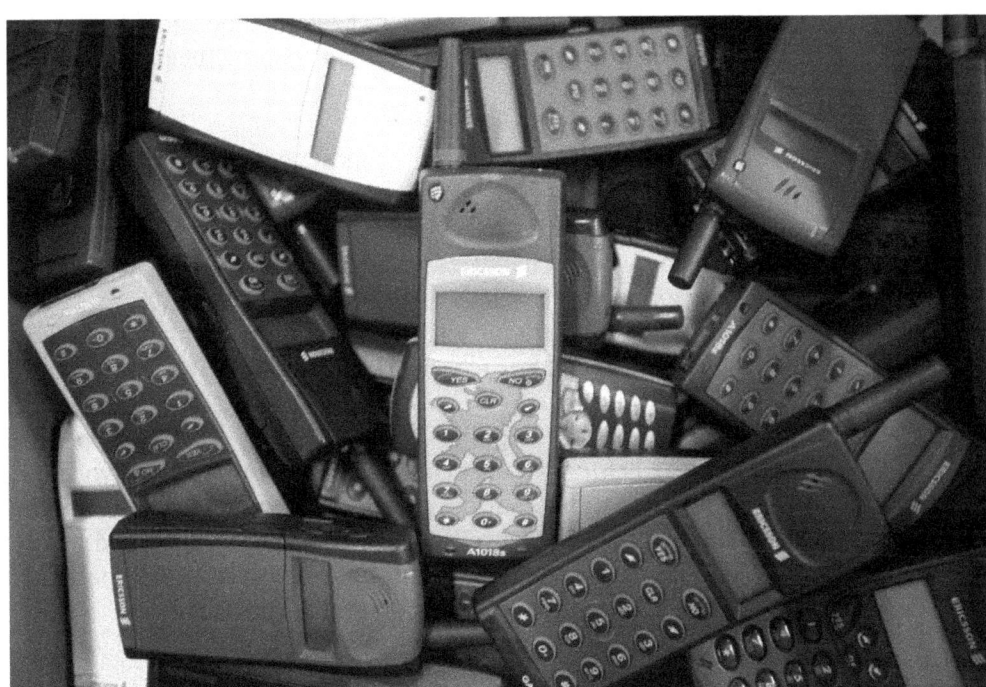

Mobile services

When you choose a mobile service the most important thing to [consider] is how you expect to use your mobile phone. First answer the following questions:
- How often will you use your phone?
- At what time of the day will you make most of your [calls]?
- Which mobile network is used by most of the people you are [likely] to call?
- What kind of [services] do you want on your mobile (for example mobile internet services)?
- Will you make much use of the more [expensive] types of calls, such as calls to [premium rate] services or using your phone [whilst] [abroad]?
- Which networks have ['coverage'] (give a good signal) where you will use your mobile?

There are so many mobile services and prices change so [often] that any [detailed] [summary] or price [comparisons] would quickly be [out of date]. The best deal [depends] on each [customer's] needs and [usage pattern] – so [general] advice could be [misleading].

But there are ways to compare prices. Before you buy, it helps if you have some idea of your general [usage], perhaps from old telephone bills. You could then have a look in [independent] magazines or find more information on websites. These generally provide up-to-date prices and detailed [assessments] of [handsets].

The next thing to do is to find out what standards of service are offered by mobile phone companies. You can find out more about network coverage from:
- mobile phone companies' websites (where you can check detailed [factual] information on coverage by postcode);
- mobile phone shops;
- Oftel's website.

For [figures] on calls [connected] and [completed] on each network for each UK region, see consumer information section at www.oftel.gov.uk/consumer/advice.

There are three [main] ways to pay. Each method should offer you a choice of [tariffs] so you can select the one that best [suits] your [needs].

Monthly contract:
- You are [billed] for calls and monthly [subscriptions], typically for a minimum contract period of at least 12 months.
- There is a wider choice of services and handsets.
- Call charges and handsets are generally cheaper.
- You normally get inclusive call minutes, for example an [allowance] of [call minutes] (and perhaps also text messages) which is included in your monthly subscription and not [charged] for [separately].

Prepay (or 'pay as you go'):
- You pay before making calls, for example with a call [voucher].
- Unlike a monthly contract, there are no credit checks or minimum contract period.
- There is usually a more [limited] choice of services and handsets.
- It is easy to control [spending], but you will not get a specified bill and call charges tend to be higher than with a monthly contract.

Pay [up front]:
- You are billed monthly, so you can see where your money is going.
- You are not charged monthly subscriptions.
- Call charges and the price and range of handsets are similar to prepay.

Apart from choosing the right mobile phone company and tariff for your usage pattern, you might find it useful to consider what it costs to call people on other networks.

Often you will pay more to call someone on a different mobile network than to call someone on the same network. On [average], you pay over three times as much, but the difference can be even bigger, especially outside [peak times]. You may be able to save money by choosing a tariff where the inclusive call minutes cover all networks, not just your network. Charges for calling different networks do not [vary] much. Besides the network coverage it is important to find out what is included within the monthly contract. You should find out exactly what you can get for your money:
- Do inclusive call minutes cover calls to people on other networks as well as yours?
- Do you get inclusive text messages and/or mobile internet call time?
- Is voicemail free of charge?
- Can you buy extra services to save money, for example [cheaper] [rates] for text messages or calls to other networks?
- For how long will any [unused] inclusive call minutes in one month be [carried forward]?

– Can you use more than one handset on the same account? (Normally this involves a relatively low extra monthly [fee], and a different phone number for each handset.)

Questions about the text

Answer the following questions about the text.

1. What is the most important thing to find out when you choose a mobile service?

2. What do you want to know about the places where you would like to use your phone?

3. What does the text say about mobile services and prices?

4. How can you get the best deal for you?

5. What can you learn from old telephone bills?

6. Where can you find information about network coverage?

7. In what ways can you pay for your mobile service?

8. For how long do you have to pay when you have a monthly contract?

9. How do you pay when you use a prepay phone?

10. How much more do you usually have to pay to call someone on a different mobile network?

4.2
Listening Skills 6

I HAVE BEEN ROBBED!

Angela (A) bought and paid for a TV and VCR in a department store. These [items] were to be delivered to her home. However, that never happened. Listen to the conversation that she has on the phone with someone from customer's service (C).

C: Customer's service, can I help you?

A: Hello, this is Angela Robinson speaking. Four weeks ago I bought a television and VCR set from your shop. I expected the set to be delivered to my house yesterday, but no such luck. I called the store to inquire after the [delivery] and they assured me that it was on its way. However, it still has not arrived. So I went back to the store and they told me that there would be no more deliveries this week! I would be the first on their list next Tuesday after the [bank holiday] [break]. But I told them I had to work that day and so I asked them to come on Wednesday.

C: And did they do that Ms. Robinson?

A: No, they [apparently] decided to come on Tuesday anyway, because when I phoned them on Wednesday after having waited all day they told me it had been delivered and left with a neighbour within my block of flats on the day before. I was informed of who this neighbour is and I went to find out if the neighbour had indeed received the items. He claims to know nothing about any delivery.

C: Oh dear, I can understand why you are so upset. Did you contact the store again after that?

A: Yes I did. I spoke to the sales manager, a lady called Ms. Heriot. She kept telling me that they were looking into matters and that they would get in touch with me when they knew more.

C: I presume that's what she did?

A: After I called several times, I was refered to the [store manager] Mr. Young. He assured me that they were still investigating the [whereabouts] of my goods. And I have still no [telly]!

C: Did Mr. Young not get back to you [either] then?

A: I made several calls and visits to the store and each time I met with indifference and [annoyance] on the part of the store staff. They were treating me as if I were at [fault], while this entire situation has been brought about by negligence and [incompetence] on their part. The last thing that they said was that they had done their part by making the delivery and that they had proof of delivery to [support] this. It was now up to me to [report] the neighbour in question to the police for the [theft] of goods.

C: This is very important. Are you sure you did not give them your neighbour's address?

A: Of course I didn't do that. Otherwise I wouldn't be so angry! I am still [struggling] to get all this [resolved] and I feel I have no rights whatsover as a [consumer].

C: Please try to stay calm Ms. Heriot. I'm sure we can work this all out. Now lets just start from the beginning...

Idioms

Vertaal de volgende woorden uit het gesprek:

1. videorecorder –
2. warenhuis –
3. afleveren –
4. klantenservice –
5. informatie vragen –
6. verzekeren –
7. beweert –
8. overstuur –
9. verkoopleider/directeur –
10. de zaak onderzoeken –
11. contact opnemen –
12. aannemen –
13. doorverwijzen naar –
14. onderzoeken –
15. goederen –
16. terugkomen op –
17. onverschilligheid –
18. aan de kant van –
19. nalatigheid –
20. bewijs –

4.3 Research

Shopping on the Internet

The increasing [availability] of the internet and digital TV means that it's now even easier to shop without leaving your home. But as a consumer, you should still take care when paying for goods and services.
The following website: http://www.consumerdirect.gov.uk/general/internet/fs_so1.shtml provides information on the following subjects:
- before you buy;
- paying for goods online;
- what do to if things go wrong;
- internet [auctions];
- where to go for help.

Assignment

1 Ga naar de website die genoemd wordt en kies twee van de onderwerpen uit het rijtje.
2 Schrijf in het Engels op wat er gezegd wordt over het onderwerp.
3 Geef daarna in tweetallen advies aan elkaar over het onderwerp dat je gekozen

Foto: Paul van Riel/
Hollandse Hoogte

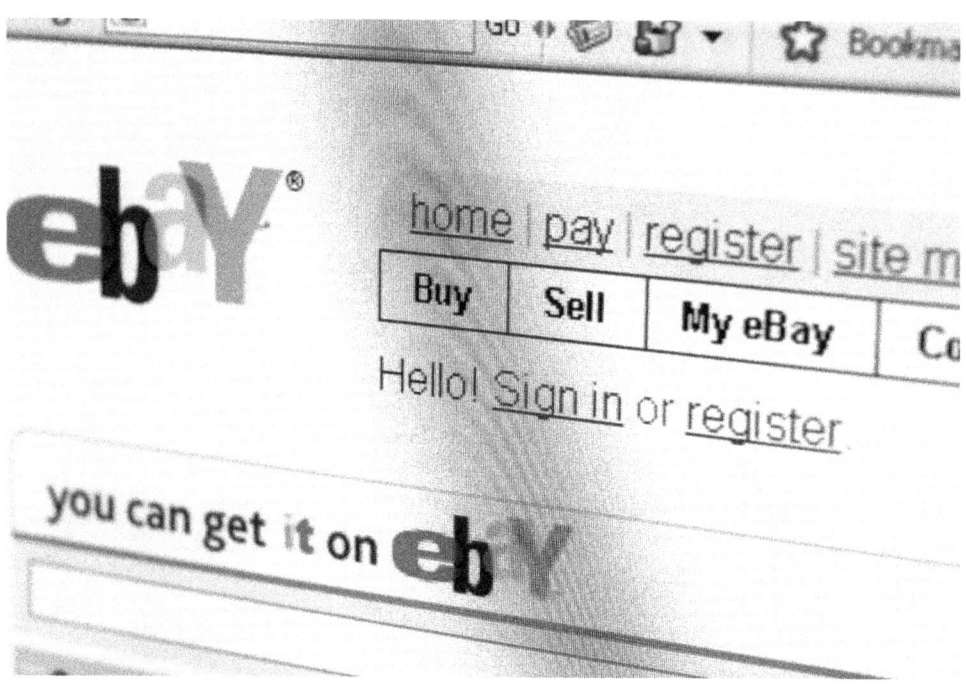

hebt. Probeer hierbij zo veel mogelijk verschillende onderwerpen aan bod te laten komen.

4.4 Grammar: Questions and negations

Wanneer je een zin **vragend** of **ontkennend** wil maken, kijk je eerst of er een hulpwerkwoord in de zin staat zoals *to have, to be, can, could* of enkele andere.

1. Er staat een **hulpwerkwoord** in de zin.

Maak de zin **vragend** door het hulpwerkwoord vooraan de zin te zetten.

| I *am* working too hard. | – | *Are* you working too hard? |
| The patient *can* take an aspirin. | – | *Can* the patient take an aspirin? |

Maak de zin *ontkennend* door **not** achter het hulpwerkwoord te zetten.

| Peter *is* complaining about her | – | Peter *is not* complaining about her. |
| I *could* use some warm clothes. | – | I *could not* use some warm clothes. |

2. Er staat **geen hulpwerkwoord** in de zin.

Maak de zin *vragend* met behulp van het werkwoord **do** of **does**.

| I *feel* awful today. | – | *Do* you *feel* awful today? |
| Toby *walks* with a limp. | – | *Does* Toby *walk* with a [limp]? |

Maak de zin *ontkennend* door **do not (don't)** of **does not (doesn't)** voor het werkwoord te zetten.

You *ask* too much. — You *do not* (don't) ask too much.
The man *needs* help. — The man *does not* (doesn't) need help.

Let op!
De **-s** achter *need* valt weg in de ontkennende zin.

Exercise

Vertaal de zinnen. Maak ze daarna (a.) vragend en (b.) ontkennend.
Bijvoorbeeld:

Sheila is ziek. Sheila is ill.
a Is Sheila ill?
b Sheila is not ill.

1. De patiënt voelt zich misselijk.

a

b

2. De kinderen verstoppen zich onder het bureau.

a

b

3. De oude vrouw begrijpt waar ik het over heb.

a

b

4. De dokter loopt de spreekkamer binnen.

a

b

5. Justin maakt vanmiddag zijn administratie af.

a

b

6. Marjory kan je vertellen hoe je haar moet aanpakken.

a

b

7. Ian vindt zijn werk erg leuk.

a

b

8. Het meisje heeft geen ouders meer.

a

b

9. Oudere mensen lopen langzamer dan jongere mensen.

a

b

10. Jez heeft alles klaargemaakt voor de volgende vergadering.

a

b

4.5 Translation

Exercise

Translate the following sentences.

1. Waar heeft u pijn?

2. Wat is er aan de hand?

3. Vertel me wat er gebeurd is.

4. Heeft u vaak last van tandpijn?

5. Wanneer bent u behandeld?

4.6 Writing

Product information

Think of three products you would really like to buy. Try to find out as much as you can about these products (Internet, magazines) and fill in the details.

Product 1	Product 2	Product 3	Name of the product
Price			
Model or type			
Colour			
Power system			
Use			
[Guarantee]			
[Waste disposal fee]			
[Method of payment]			

4.7 Speaking

Foto: Willem Mes/ Hollandse Hoogte

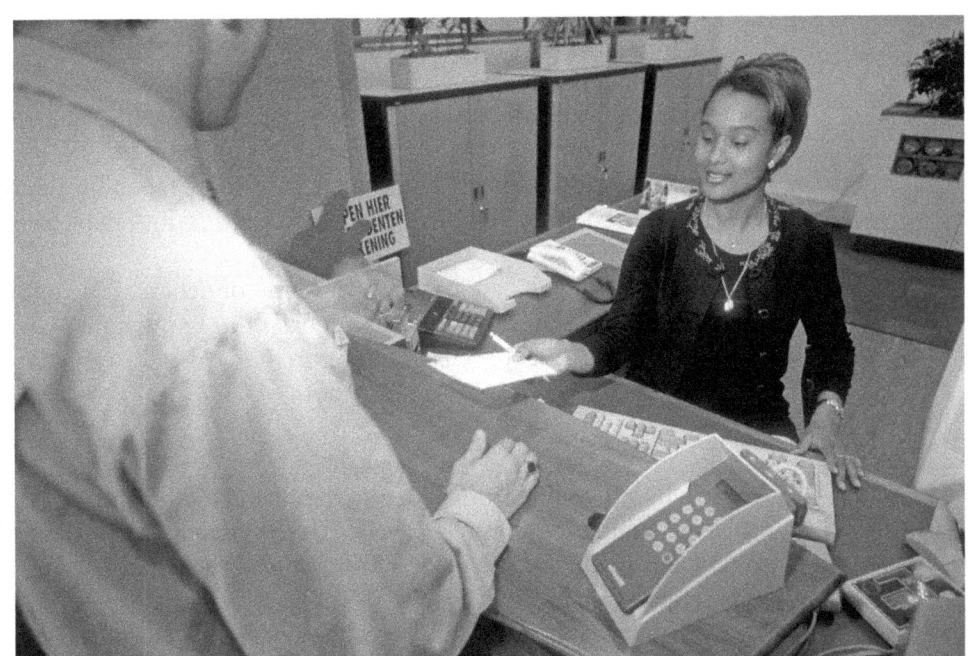

RETURN YOUR PRODUCT

Imagine you bought one of the products from the previous exercise. When the product is delivered at your house you find out you are not happy with it. You are going to make a phone call in which you [demand] that the product will be [collected] again.

Practice this roleplay with another student. One student is the caller and the other student someone from customer's service. Take turns in the different roles.

When you are the caller:
Think of a number of reasons why you are not happy with the product. Examples are:
- You have to pay more than you agreed on.
- It doesn't work properly.
- It's the wrong colour / model /type.
- It doesn't fit in your house.
- You can't pay for it.
- You don't like it anymore.

When you are the customer's service person:
Think of a number of reasons why the other person cannot return the product. Examples are:
- The product or it's wrapping has been opened.
- The customer waited too long.
- There are no other colours / models /types [available].
- The customer has signed an agreement.
- It seems like the customer ruined the product him/herself.

4.8
Reading

Are you [in debt]?

TOO YOUNG TO BE IN DEBT?

If you are under 18, you can't apply for credit cards, [overdrafts] and personal [loans]. That said, you could [fall into debt] in other ways, such as [borrowing] money from your friends or your parents.
If you're struggling [to make ends meet] and you're [spending] more money than you [earn], you need to do something about it. Getting into debt could [affect] you for years to come.
No matter how old you are or what your level of debt is, it's important to understand how debt can [mount up]. It's also important to know how to deal with debt problems if you ever [face] them in the future.

[RECOGNISING] DEBT

People who are in debt [often] make the mistake of [ignoring] the size of the problem, hoping it will just go away. [Unfortunately], debt has a [habit] of hanging around and getting worse, so it's important to recognise the [warning signs] at an early stage.
If you're always short on cash, or you're constantly close to your overdraft limit on your [bank account], then you should think about taking some action [straight away].

Ask yourself where you'd find the money if you had to make a big payment [at short notice] or in an [emergency]. If the answer is simply [extending] your overdraft, then you could be in danger of getting into serious debt.

DOING SOMETHING ABOUT IT

The earlier you start to [tackle] the problem, the easier it will be. If your financial situation is in danger of becoming serious, do something about it now.
The worst thing you can do if you're having money problems is to just [ignore] the situation. It's often the case that people [assume] they'll be able to pay off their debt in the future when they start earning more money.
But anything could happen. [Interest charges] and late payment [fees] could mean that you're faced with a debt that's a lot more than you expected - sometimes double the amount you originally [owed].

WHAT YOU CAN DO

If you are in debt, it might be that you've lost [grasp] of your finances. For example, do you know exactly how much money goes in and out of your bank account and how often?
You can make a start by looking at your recent [bank statements] and finding out where you are spending money on things you could easily do without. By getting rid of these, your [cash flow] situation will get better quite quickly.
If your situation is a bit more serious and you owe money to a number of people or companies, you'll need to start planning a budget and organising your various debts. Once you know exactly how many debts you have and the total of each one, you can prioritise the most important ones and start to pay them off.

Exercise

Read the text and then write in your own words:

1. What says the first paragraph about age and debt?

2. What says the text about when you should do something about your debts?

3. What can you do according to the text?

4. Zet de woorden uit de tekst bij de woorden met dezelfde betekenis

emergency –

straight away –

overdraft –

to earn –

to tackle –

to mount up –

at short notice –

fees –

to owe –

cash flow –

Woorden met dezelfde betekenis:
- with little warning
- amount of money being transferred
- to deal with
- unexpected dangerous situation
- immediately
- money paid for services
- an excess of money spent
- have an obligation to pay
- to obtain money for work
- to become larger

4.9 Grammar: Personal and Possessive Pronouns

Personal and *Possessive Pronouns* (persoonlijke en bezittelijke voornaamwoorden) in het Engels:

	1	2	3	4
ik	I	me	my	mine
jij	you	you	your	yours
hij	he	him	his	his
zij	she	her	her	hers
het	it	it	its	its
wij	we	us	our	ours
jullie	you	you	your	yours
zij	they	them	their	theirs

Lijst **1** gebruik je wanneer het voornaamwoord het **onderwerp** in de zin is.

Ik werk hier graag. — *I* like working here.

Lijst **2** gebruik je wanneer het voornaamwoord het **lijdend voorwerp** in de zin is.

Hij belde *mij*. — He called *me*.

Lijst **3** gebruik je wanneer je het voornaamwoord **voor een zelfstandig naamwoord** gebruikt.

Het is *mijn* boek. — It is *my* book.

Lijst **4** gebruik je na van.

Het boek is *van mij*. — The book is *mine*.

Exercise

Geef telkens de goede Engelse vorm.
1 The woman ran into the room saying that it was _____ (haar) bag, but the bag was not _____ (van haar).
2 Excuse me, is this _____ (uw) prescription or is it _____ (van mij)?
3 _____ (hij) always asks _____ (haar) about _____ (haar) health.
4 The patients are talking about _____ (hun) complaints.
5 _____ (zij) is the one who took _____ (onze) magazines
6 Is this _____ (zijn) wheelchair? No, it is _____ (van hem).
7 Don't forget _____ (uw) medication. It is _____ (van u), isn't it?
8 _____ (het) isn't _____ (mijn) fault! Why do _____ (jij) always blame _____ (mij)?

4.10 Writing

Numbers

Write the following numbers [in full].

Example: 10	ten	tiende	10th	tenth
0	nought, zero	–	–	–
1		eerste		
2		tweede		
3		derde		
4		vierde		
5		vijfde		

Example: 10	ten	tiende	10th	tenth
6		zesde		
7		zevende		
8		achtste		
9		negende		
11		elfde		
12		twaalfde		
13		dertiende		
20		twintigste		
21		eenentwintig-ste		
100		honderdste		
200		tweehonderd-ste		
1000		eenduizendste		
1.000.000		eenmiljoenste		

5 How to survive my norms and values?

5.1 Reading

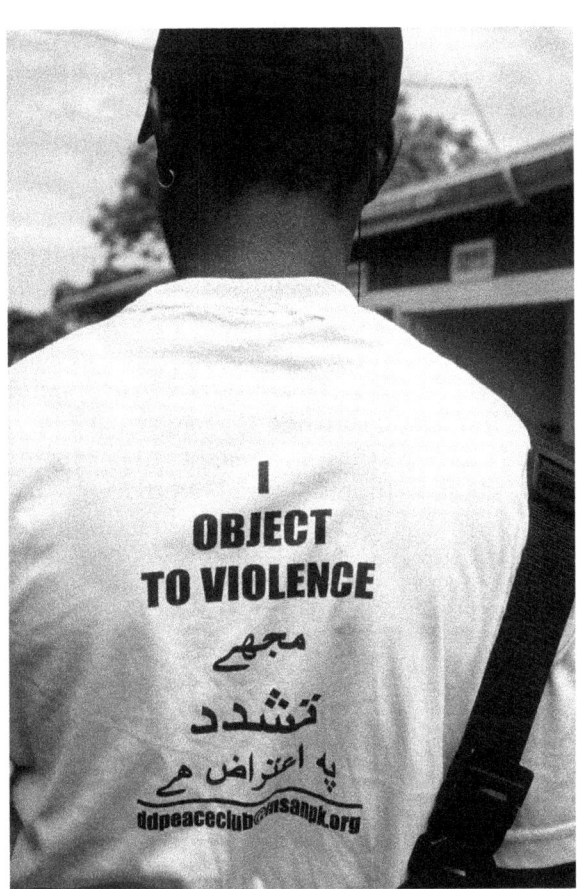

Foto: Roel Burger/
Hollandse Hoogte

Do we need [citizenship]?

The term citizenship [refers to] you as an individual who is not only part of a [certain] country or state but it looks a bit further than that. It offers a new way of thinking on how we live together and includes the idea of 'status' and 'role'. Citizenship [involves] [issues] relating to [rights and duties], but also ideas of equality, [diversity] and social justice. It concerns the individual and his/her relations with others.
A [fundamental] aim is the promotion of a culture of democracy and human rights, a culture that [enables] individuals to develop and build communities. In order for this to happen social [cohesion], [mutual understanding] and solidarity needs to be strengthened.
Citizenship is aimed at all individuals, [regardless] of their [age] or role in society. It

helps [pupils], young people and adults participate actively, and responsibly in the [decision-making] processes in their communities. Participation is the [key] to the promotion and strengthening of a democratic culture based on [awareness] and [commitment] to shared [fundamental values], such as human rights and freedoms and the [rule of law].

It is based on the idea that individuals construct themselves and their relationships [in accordance with] certain values. The values held by an individual can change. These values can influence how an individual makes decisions. They make it easier to choose and help to structure the environment.

Special attention is given to those values that [underpin] the idea of democracy and human rights. These include: recognition of and respect for oneself and others, the [ability] to listen, and to [engage] in peaceful conflict [resolution].

It is important that people know about the rules of collective life and how these rules developed, their origin and their [purpose]. It is also important that learners have an understanding of the levels of power within society and how public institutions work. In order to be able to understand a democratic society you need to be able to understand 'the world'. The world is in a [constant] state of change. To [participate] actively in the [development] of society, people need to have some knowledge of the debates of our time, for example: what is meant by cultural rights? What do we mean by responsibility?

Citizenship aims to improve people's ability to take initiative and to accept responsibilities in society. These are the [capacities] that [empower] the individual to take an active part in and contribute to the community, in the shaping of its [affairs] and in solving problems.

There is the clear recognition that knowledge, [attitudes] and values only take on meaning in everyday personal and social life. Such capacities include: the capacity to live and work with one another, to co-operate, to engage in joint initiatives, to be able to [resolve] conflicts in a [non-violent] manner and to take part in public debates.

The concept of 'responsibilities' [implies] the ability to [respond] – being [responsive to] others, and being [responsible] for oneself. The idea of responsibility applies to governments on the one hand and to individuals on the other.

Questions about the text

1. *citizenship* in line 1 refers to:
a being a nation or state
b to live in the city
c being a citizen of a particular country
d being part of Europe

2. *equality* in line 4 refers to:
a being the same in status, right and opportunities
b being a bit more equal than others
c being different from others
d being responsible for others

3. *justice* in line 5 refers to:
a being right
b being wrong
c being [unfair] and [unreasonable]
d being [fair] and reasonable

4. *communities* in line 7 refers to:
a people traveling around
b people who don't live at home

c group of people who own everything
d groups of people living together in one place

5. *solidarity* in line 8 refers to:
a [mutual] support within a group
b being firm or strong
c self-centred, egoism
d [reliance] on one's own strength

6. *collective* in line 23 refers to:
a a group of things
b done by people acting as a group
c done by individuals
d on one's own

7. An example of a public institution is a:
a house.
b market.
c public toilet.
d school.

8. Another word for *debate* in line 29 is:
a discussion.
b argument.
c story.
d definition.

9. *to contribute* in line 33 means:
a ask something
b give in order to help
c collect money
d to pay money for a club

10. A joint initiative
a is something you do when asked.
b is something you develop alone.
c is something you come up with together.
d is something you do by yourself.

5.2
Listening Skills 7

Private and [professional attitude]

An interviewer is [engaged in] a conversation with 3 people who work in the health service. The topic of discussion is the difference between private and professional attitude. The interviewer (I) speaks with Jacky (J) who works in a day-care centre for children, Paul (P) who works as a socio-cultural worker in a community centre and Anissa (A) who works as a nurse in a health centre.

I: Welcome all. The issue that I would like to address this morning is whether we behave differently at work [compared to] at home and if we do so, how? Who would like to start?

J: I don't think you are a completely different person at work, but I do treat my own children different from the children in my playgroup at work.

I: Can you give me an example of this then?

J: Well I can't lose my temper at work when a child does something naughty. But when my daughter does the same thing over and over, I sometimes snap at her.

P: Are you saying you never lose your self-control at work? I know I do sometimes.

I: What happens then?

P: Well I have these contracts with the youngsters that come to the centre. For some of them it's their last chance to make something of their life. If they are deliberately [messing that up] I just lose my patience sometimes and give up.

A: But do you never lose your patience at home?

P: With my wife you mean? No that's quite different.

I: What makes your home situation different from your professional situation?

P: It's the nature of the relationship that [matters]. At work you have a [functional relation] and my relation at home is based more on love and intimacy.

I: Can anyone see an overlap between the two?

A: For me, the main thing in any relationship is respect. Both at home and at work. If you respect the other person, then you can [accomplish] anything really.

J: Yes, respect is an important aspect but I would like to add trust. That is important in every relationship too. If there's no trust, then there is no basis for anything. The parents that bring their children to our centre have to trust us to treat their children well. The children are still so small that they can't stand up for themselves.

P: I find abuse of trust one of the most difficult things in my job. It's really hard sometimes to give someone yet another chance after he has [betrayed] your trust. I'm not quite sure I would give my friends as many chances as that. So maybe it has to do with expectations as well. At work you don't expect as much, because otherwise you can't do your job.

A: May be you are right, but when I give parents advice on their child's diet I do expect them to follow that.

P: Yes, of course you do and you should. But you would still help them even if they didn't take your advice, wouldn't you?

I: Are you saying you accept more from others at work?

P: I [suppose] so.

I: So what we have heard is that there are differences and similarities in your attitude at home and at work and that expectations play an important role. Thank you all for your comments. I think this is a subject that we could discuss for hours but unfortunately our time is up.

Idioms

Vertaal de volgende woorden uit het gesprek:

1. houding –
2. gesprek –
3. gespreksonderwerp –
4. verschil –
5. kinderdagverblijf –
6. peuterklas –

7. boos worden –
8. ondeugend –
9. snauwen –
10. opzettelijk –
11. mijn geduld verliezen –
12. aard –
13. intimiteit –
14. toevoegen –
15. voor zichzelf opkomen –
16. misbruik van vertrouwen –
17. verwachtingen –
18. houding –
19. opmerkingen –
20. helaas –

5.3 Speaking

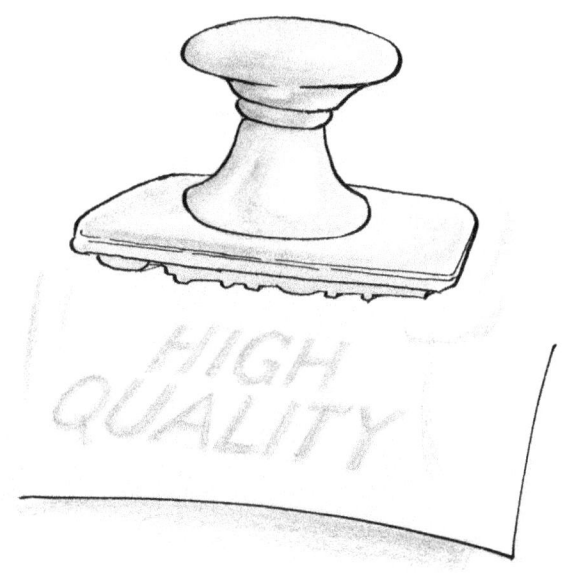

HOW TO IMPROVE THE [QUALITY OF LIFE]

In your life and [environment] there are always things that could be better. In this exercise you have to think of and present a number of ideas that could improve your quality of life. This can be at home, at school or in your work place.
You work in pairs. One student presents the new ideas, the other student listens and reacts.

[POINTERS] FOR THE SPEAKER

– Write down in a few words what you are going to say.
– Try to stay centred in your presentation.
– Use body language.

- Offer factual information.
- Check if the listener understands what you are saying.
- Give examples when necessary.
- Underline the [ethical value] of the matter.
- Try to convince the listener.

POINTERS FOR THE LISTENER

- Listen carefully to the speaker.
- Ask for factual information.
- Do not interrupt the speaker.

EXAMPLES OF SUBJECTS

- [prejudice] on the work floor (women can't be managers etc);
- equal pay for men and women;
- homework;
- pocketmoney;
- the amount of [overtime];
- bullying.

5.4 Grammar: the Present Perfect Tense

De *Present Perfect Tense* (voltooid tegenwoordige tijd) wordt gevormd door **have/has** en het **voltooid deelwoord** (zie appendix A).

I have done
He/she/it has finished
We/you/they have lost

De Present Perfect Tense wordt in het Nederlands op twee manieren vertaald: VTT *of* al + OTT.

VTT

| Peter has broken his leg. | – | Peter **heeft** zijn been **gebroken**. |

al + OTT

| I *have worked* in a youth centre **since 1990**. | – | Ik **werk al** sinds 1990 in een jeugdcentrum. |

Deze vorm geeft het volgende aan:
1. Het verwijst naar een niet nader gedefinieerd verleden.

| *Have* you *ever given* him advice? | – | Heb je hem ooit advies gegeven? |
| *I've worked* there only once. | – | Ik heb daar maar één keer gewerkt. |

2. Iets is in het verleden gebeurd en heeft nu nog effect.

The girl *has lost* her mother.	–	Het meisje is haar moeder verloren.
The officer in charge *has gone* home.	–	De dienstdoende agent is naar huis gegaan.

3. Iets is in het verleden begonnen en duurt nu nog voort, met vermelding van de tijdsduur.

I *haven't seen* a doctor since last week.	–	Ik heb sinds vorige week geen dokter meer gezien.
She *has lived* with this disease for 15 years.	–	Ze heeft deze ziekte al 15 jaar.

Exercise

Zet het woord tussen haakjes in de goede vorm. Gebruik hierbij Appendix A.
1 I _____ his name. (*forget*)
2 He _____ already _____. (*go*)
3 I _____ it up yet. (*look up*)
4 She _____ up smoking. (*give up*)
5 He _____ an appointment. (*make*)

5.5
Translation

Exercise

Translate the following sentences.
1. We zijn open van 9 uur 's morgens tot 6 uur 's avonds.

2. U moet eerst een afspraak maken.

3. U kunt hier geen medicijnen krijgen.

4. Als de klachten erger worden, moet u ons terugbellen.

5. Wie is uw verhuurder?

5.6
Writing

Programme for [exchange students]

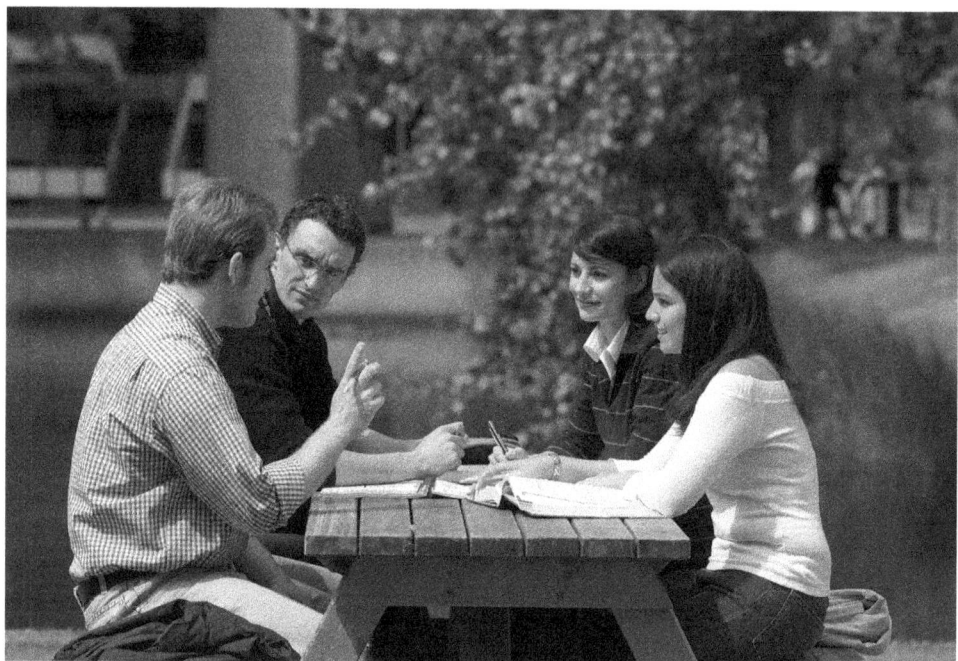

Ronald van den Heerik/Hollandse Hoogte

Een aantal Zweedse studenten komt binnenkort voor een uitwisseling naar jouw school. Er moet een aantal dingen worden georganiseerd zoals:
- een introductiebijeenkomst;
- een rondleiding door de school;
- een rondleiding op de werk / stageplek;
- een gezamenlijke lunch;
- een korte wandeling door de woonplaats;
- een feestavond.

Er is afgesproken dat Engels de voertaal is.

Exercise

1. Make [pairs] and choose one of the activities mentioned.

2. Write down in English what you are going to do and how. Describe:
- what the activity is all about;
- where to meet and how to get there;
- how many people are going together;
- who will coordinate the activity;
- if the students need anything to [prepare] themselves.

3. Write down all the things you need:
- people;
- materials, food, drinks;
- transport;
- money;

- where and how you are going to get the things you need.

4. Write an invitation for the students. The invitation should mention:
- what the activity is all about;
- the time (start and finish);
- the place ([map]);
- the things they need to bring;
- what they can expect.

5.7 Reading and research

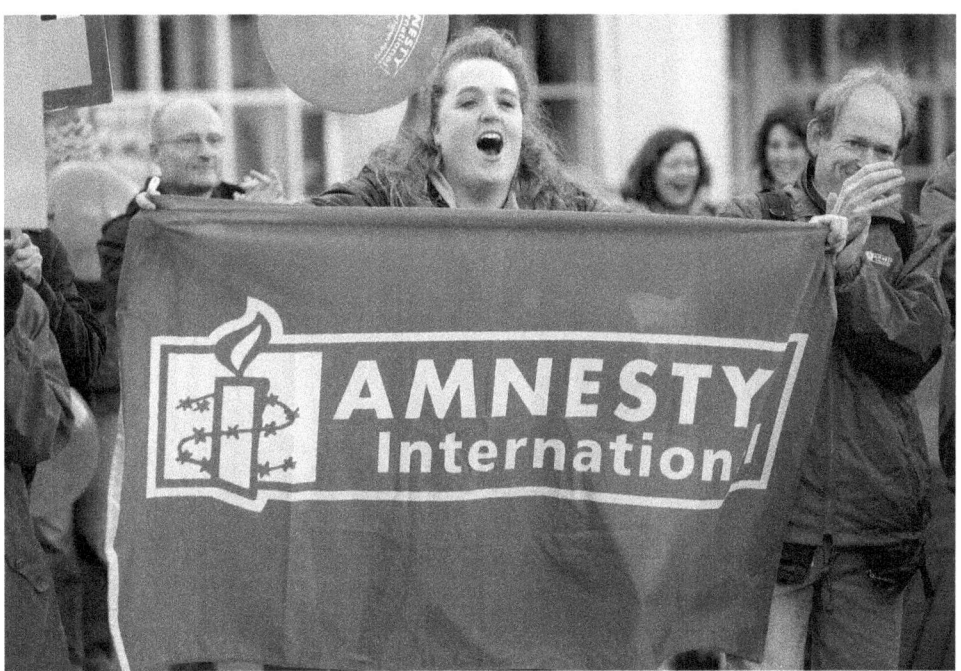

Foto: Arie Kievit/ Hollandse Hoogte

About Amnesty International

Amnesty International is a worldwide [movement] of people who campaign for internationally [recognized] human rights.

The movement's vision is of a world in which every person [enjoys] all of the human rights as [determined] in the [Universal Declaration] of Human Rights and other international human rights [agreements].

The mission of Amnesty International is to [undertake] research and action [focused on] [preventing] and ending [grave] [physical or mental] [abuses], protecting [freedom of expression], and to protect against discrimination, within the context of its work to [promote] all human rights.

Amnesty International is [independent] of any [government], political [ideology], [economic interest] or religion. It does not support or [oppose] any government or political system, nor does it support or oppose the [views] of the [victims] whose rights it [seeks] to [protect]. It is [concerned] [solely] with the [impartial] protection of human rights.

Amnesty International has a varied network of members and supporters around the world. At the latest [count], there were more than 1.8 million [members], supporters and [subscribers] in over 150 countries in every region of the world. [Although] they come from many different [backgrounds] and have widely different political and religious [beliefs], they are [united] by a [determination] to work for a world where everyone enjoys human rights.

To do:
- Go to: 'Campaigns' or 'Act now' on their website.
- Choose one of the campaigns that are mentioned.
- Download or print one of the letters.
- If you want to write a letter yourself you can use the: 'Letter writing guide'.
- You can send the letter or bring a printed copy to class.
- Discuss with other students why you chose the campaign you did and compare your letters.

5.8 Listening Skills 8

Flight from Vietnam

Listen to the following conversation that a reporter (R) has with Nguyen (N), a refugee from Vietnam.

R: Welcome in the studio Nguyen. You have asked to be [identified] only by your family name. Why is that?

N: I am still scared they will pick me up and bring me back to Vietnam. I also don't want to endanger other refugees.

R: Can you tell us about yourself? You are 36 now and live in the state of Virginia in the United States. Why did you decide to leave Vietnam?

N: I decided to leave after I was [refused] entry into [college], [despite] passing the entrance exams. The reason they refused me was the fact that my father had been an officer in the South Vietnamese military. At that point, I thought I had to leave because there was no future there for me. I passed the test for the college and still they won't accept me just because of my family background.

R: So how did you [flee]? Can you tell us something about your journey?

N: There were only two ways for me to leave the country, both [risky]. I could walk to Cambodia, but it was very dangerous. Even if I made it to Cambodia, the next challenge would be to get into Thailand, which is not under [Communist rule]. Leaving by boat was the obvious choice. It was a dark night. We had to go through the jungle to get to the boat waiting outside. I was very frightened.

R: Did you have to pay to get on this boat?

N: My family paid U.S. $1500. We all [quietly] boarded a small boat that took us to a larger boat that was waiting out to sea. It was to take us away from Vietnam. For safety's sake, the boat had [to appear] to anyone who saw it as if it were only a fishing boat. All of the refugees, more than 120, had to stay [hidden] below [deck]. There was no room to stand up. We were forced [to curl] into a fetal position.

R: How long did that journey last?

N: We had to stay that way for three days, the time it took to leave Vietnam's [territorial waters]. It was horrible. We never experienced that before, we'd never been out to sea. I was almost dead... There were too many people, [crammed into] one place. The waves were so big.

R: I can imagine. What happened next?

N: After leaving Vietnam's maritime border, the boat met calmer seas and passengers were permitted outside the [hold]. They could get fresh air, but little else. There was no food or water because of some miscommunication. Occasionally, we got lucky. A big ship would sometimes pass by and throw us whatever water and food they had. We lived like that for 21 days until we got to Malaysia. The Malaysian [navy] gave us a bigger boat, food, water, and a compass so that we would know which direction to go, to get to Indonesia. In Indonesia, we were taken to a refugee camp at Galang.

R: How do you feel about those still in Vietnam?

N: [Nowadays], the people who arrive at the camps aren't refugees, but asylum-seekers. I feel sorry for them. They don't have the [opportunity] to [improve] themselves. I'm sorry they don't have freedom.

R: Some 250,000 Vietnamese lived in the refugee camp from 1976 to 1996, before being sent to Australia, Canada, Switzerland, and the United States. By the time Nguyen arrived, Vietnamese refugees were no longer automatically [granted] entry into other countries. [Proving] his status as a political refugee was easier for Nguyen than for most. He had a letter stating that he had passed his exams and was eligible for college, and the letter stating why he wasn't [allowed] to enroll at college. Even so, Nguyen spent three years in Indonesia before being screened, approved, and sent to the United States.

Bron: RFA 2025 M Street NW, Suite 300, Washington DC 20036, USA

idioms

Vertaal de volgende woorden uit het gesprek:

1. Vlucht   –
2. Vluchteling   –
3. Bang   –
4. In gevaar brengen –
5. Toegang   –
6. toelatingsexamen –
7. Achtergrond   –
8. Reis   –
9. Gevaarlijk   –
10. Uitdaging   –
11. Beste keuze   –
12. Aan boord gaan –
13. Om veiligheidsredenen –
14. Foetushouding   –
15. vreselijk   –
16. Golven   –
17. Toegestaan   –
18. soms   –
19. Vluchtelingenkamp –
20. Asielzoekers   –
21. In aanmerking komen voor –
22. Inschrijven   –

23. Doorgelicht –
24. goedgekeurd –
25. Amerika –

5.9 Grammar: Relative Pronouns

Relative Pronouns (betrekkelijke voornaamwoorden) kunnen verwijzen naar personen, dieren en dingen.

De volgende Engelse voornaamwoorden komen hier aan bod:

Enkelvoud	Meervoud		
who(m)	die, wie	dat, wat	die, wie
which	die, wie	dat, wat	die, wie
that	die, wie	dat, wat	die, wie
whose	wiens/wier (van wie)	wier	
which	wat/hetgeen	wat/hetgeen	

In het Engels gelden de volgende regels:

1. Voor **personen** wordt gebruikt: **who, who(m), whose.**

a. Who als **onderwerp** van de zin:

The man *who* lives next door is an alcoholic. – De man die hiernaast woont, is een alcholist.

b. Who(m) als lijdend of meewerkend voorwerp:

The girl *whom* I wanted to speak to was away. – Het meisje dat ik wilde spreken was weg.

Na een voorzetsel is **whom** verplicht.

The woman with *whom* he fell in love left him. – De vrouw op wie hij verliefd was geworden verliet hem.

c. Whose bij een tweede naamval:

The man *whose* wife died. – De man wiens (van wie de) vrouw overleed.

2. Voor **dieren en dingen** wordt gebruikt: **which**.

We used the medicine, *which* Anne spoke about.	–	We gebruikten het medicijn waar Anne het over gehad had.
The dog *which* bit the child was put down.	–	De hond die het kind gebeten had, werd afgemaakt.

In beperkende bijvoeglijke bijzinnen (noodzakelijke toevoeging) mag ook **that** worden gebruikt.

3. Soms wordt **that** gebruikt in plaats van **who** of **which**.

Do you know anyone *that/who* speaks Dutch?	–	Ken je iemand die Nederlands spreekt?
He works for a company *that/which* makes machines	–	Hij werkt voor een bedrijf dat machines maakt

Het voornaamwoord mag ook **weggelaten** ( ) worden; maar dit mag alleen als het betrekkelijke voornaamwoord géén onderwerp is en níet voorafgegaan wordt door een voorzetsel.

The boy ( ) the drunken driver ran over, has just died.	–	Het jongetje dat door de dronken chauffeur is overreden, is net overleden.
Is Mary the constable *that/who* warned you?	–	Is Mary de politieagent die je gewaarschuwd heeft?

Exercise

Vul het juiste betrekkelijke voornaamwoord in: who(m), which, that, whose.
1 That is the woman _____ was [raped].
2 Is that the boy to _____ you gave the medicine?
3 Do you know anyone _____ works in that [community centre]?
4 Lucy told me about her new job _____ she is enjoying very much.
5 I met a man _____ sister knows you.

5.10
Conversation

Exercise

SOCIAL NETWORK

A social network is a group of people who exchange information and contacts for professional or social [purposes]. In this exercise you first [fill in] your own social network. After that, you discuss your network with another student.

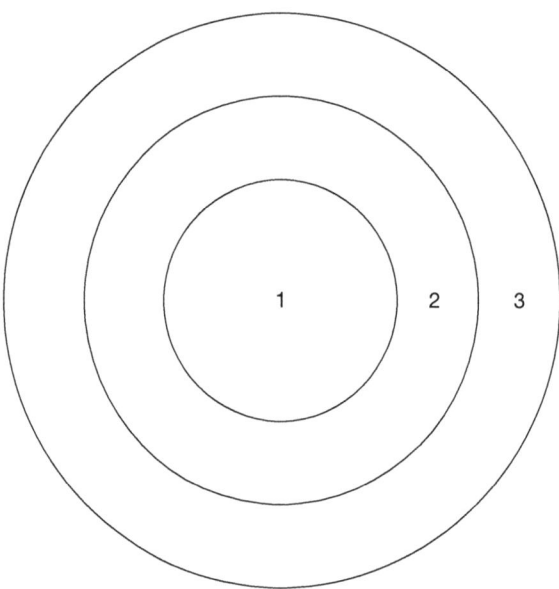

1 intimacy
2 friendship
3 [acquaintances].

[POINTERS] FOR DRAWING YOUR NETWORK

- Before you enter a name think of the circle it fits in. Your boyfriend, for example, should be placed in circle 1 and your tutor in circle 3.
- If you are not sure where to put a name you can ask yourself: what is the reason for the contact with this person? Is it emotional (comfort and support), practical (someone who gives you a lift), just for company (pub) or to give you advice and information?
- Think of how often you have contact with the people in the network.

POINTERS FOR DISCUSSING YOUR NETWORK

You can ask questions like:
- Is the network large or small?
- Has the network become smaller or bigger recently and if so why?
- Is there much variation in the network?
- Are the people in the network of a different age, [gender], culture, [marital status], education? How often does the person have contact with the people in the network in circle 1, 2, 3?
- Where do most people from the network live?
- What does the person in the network mean to or do for the student?

6 How to survive?

6.1 Reading

Read the following text.

Keeping yourself healthy

There are several things you can do yourself to keep healthy, such as eating a [balanced] diet, taking lots of [exercise] and avoiding things that damage your body such as smoking. (Never [inhale] the fumes of [substances] such as [glue]. They can damage organs and even kill.)

Different foods [contain] different substances that your body needs. These are [proteins], vitamins, minerals, water, fat, [carbohydrates] and [roughage]. The [chart] below lists the main foods in a balanced diet and explain how they help your body.

FATS

Fats [provide] more energy than carbohydrates and also vitamins, some of which you cannot get any other way.

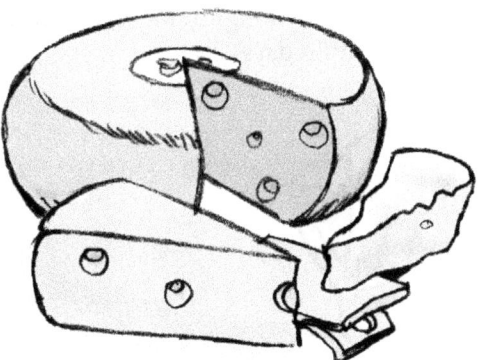

Fats.

PROTEIN

Protein is broken down and becomes [acids] called [amino acids] that your cells use for growth and to repair [tissues].

CARBOHYDRATES

Carbohydrates provide energy that you need for any physical activity. Some energy is converted into heat, [maintaining] your body temperature of 37 °C.

Protein.

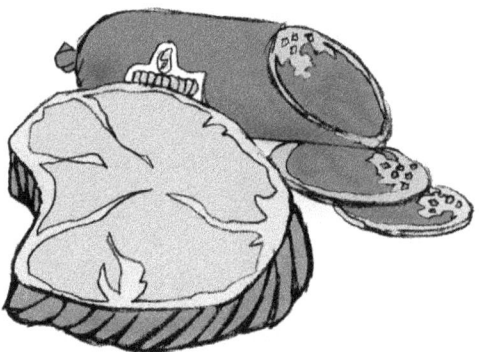

It is a good idea to exercise as much as possible to keep your body in good [working order]. Exercise helps to keep your heart pumping efficiently and keeps your [muscles] strong. It also [increases] your lung [capacity] so that more [oxygen] gets into your body. It also helps to burn off [excess] food. One of the best exercises is swimming because then you use all parts of your body [at once].

Carbohydrates.

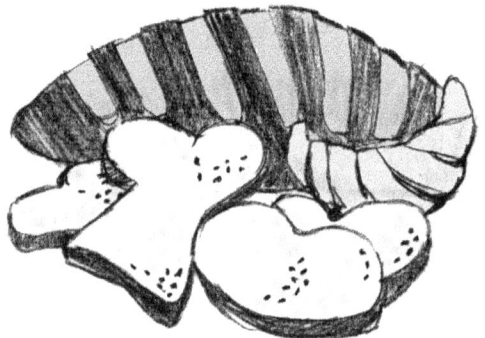

WATER

Water makes up about 70% of your [body weight]. Most food contains water. Without any food or water you would die within days.

Water.

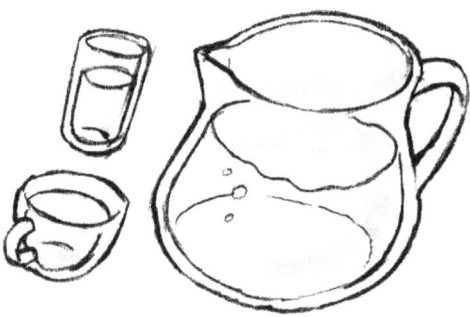

VITAMINS

Vitamins are [chemicals] that your body needs to work efficiently but cannot make itself.

Vitamins.

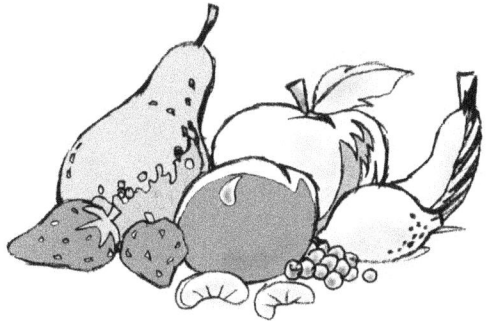

MINERALS

Minerals are used in the [construction] of [body tissues].

Minerals.

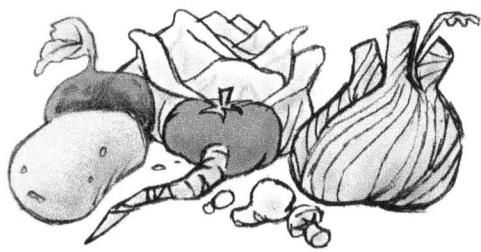

[FIBRE]

Fibre [adds] [bulk] to your diet and helps your [waste products] to keep moving.

Fibre.

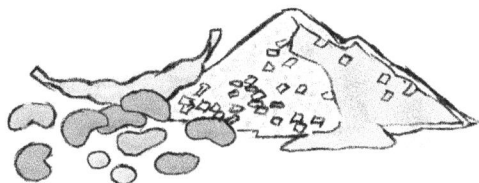

Smoking, alcohol and drugs.

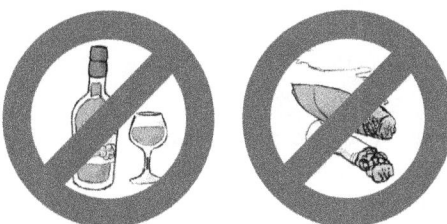

As part of preventative medicine [health workers] educate people about the effects on their bodies of smoking, alcohol and drugs. They [encourage] and help people to [avoid] these things or give them up.

Questions about the text

Read the text Food and Health in 6.1 and complete the following sentences.
1 You can keep yourself healthy by _____ .

2 Fumes of substances such as glue can _____ .
3 The different substances that our bodies need are _____ .
4 The function of fats is to _____ .
5 When protein is broken down it becomes _____ called _____ .
6 Amino acids are used by your cells for _____ .
7 _____ provide energy which you need for any physical activity.
8 Exercise helps to _____ and keeps your _____ strong.
9 Exercise increases your _____ so that more _____ gets into your body.
10 _____ are chemicals which your body needs to work efficiently but cannot make itself.
11 Minerals are used for the _____ .
12 Fibre adds bulk to your diet and helps your _____ to keep moving.
13 _____ and _____ are bad for your health.
14 _____ contain a lot of fibre.
15 _____ contain a lot of minerals.

6.2
Listening Skills 9

Healthier life

Listen to the conversation that an interviewer (I) has with Nicky (N) who has been on a journey towards a healthier lifestyle.

I: Hello Nicky. Would you like to share your [amazing] success story with us and tell how it changed your whole life?

N: Er... were shall I start? I started to gain weight when I was about 15. I don't know what happened. I wasn't obese, but I became chunky. I had a couple of bad experiences at school. People were [teasing] me, but nothing too horrible. During high school, I became much taller, pretty thin, and [fairly] active too.

I: So you had your [growth spurt].

N: Yes I did. After high school, I don't know whether it was just my [level] of physical activity that [went down], but I [gradually] seemed to gain weight. I couldn't even tell how much weight, but slowly, each year, I gained. All of a sudden, I was 22 and I was fairly big.

I: And then something happened.

N: Erm... After my boyfriend and I broke up, I changed my life completely. I went back to school and started going to the gym again, and eating well. I lost quite a bit of weight. And then, once agin, I [gradually] abandoned my workout routine, started dating Roger, and with our [opposite] [schedules], it was hard. A lot of times, I would skip the gym to go out with him. Slowly over time, the weight kind of just [crept back] up on me.

I: At this stage, Nicky weighed about 104 kg. She had reached a point where her weight was above a healthy Body Mass Index (BMI). Her weight gain had begun to affect her health. It had also affected her self-esteem...

I: Please continue your story Nicky.

N: I just wasn't happy with myself. I would sit there and say, 'I'm fat.' I hated shopping, because nothing fit. I was going to the gym, 'cause I've always liked going to the gym, but I just wasn't seeing the results I wanted to see. I knew I had to do something different. I wanted to change.

I:	And then you set a date for your marriage!	
N:	The wedding was an incentive for me. I wanted to look and feel the best I could. I had to do it for myself. I didn't even know if I would achieve my target weight by the time my wedding took place, I was hoping I would, but I wasn't being unrealistic, I thought 'If I don't make it, then I don't make it.' The wedding was a little extra push to help keep me going.	
I:	If you can't manage on your own, then you can try and find others to support you. And that is what you did isn't it Nicky?	
N:	Yes, I had tried doing it on my own for about a year. I just wasn't seeing any results. It didn't matter how often I went to the gym, month after month, it was always the same thing. I had heard good things about this support programme. I could still eat normal, everyday food. It wasn't a diet, but a lifestyle change. I learned how to pick better foods, and how to control portions. The programme also encouraged [exercise] even if it was just a little bit. I thought well, it doesn't hurt to try it.	
I:	Did you get any encouragement from the people around you?	
N:	My immediate family and my boyfriend were really supportive. I would even hear Roger talking on the phone and he'd say, 'I know her and she's going to do it. It may just be a matter of time, but she's committed.' It was very nice to hear that he believed in me. He knew I would [accomplish] my goal. People started noticing that I had lost weight, probably after I had lost about 20 pounds. Exercise was and is a release. I get to go there, it's my time. I do what I want. I put on my music, and my headphones and I go! And I like it.	
I:	Nicky reached her target weight in 9 months. Today, she is leading an active and healthy lifestyle. So how do you look back on it?	
N:	The biggest [benefit] to me is a better self-image. I feel better about myself. I still have days, like everybody, where I wake up and it doesn't matter what I put on, 'I feel fat' I am still the same person, but I think I feel more confident about myself. I like myself more and I feel better because of what I have learned.	

Bron: Based on an article by Public Health Agency of Canada

idioms

Vertaal de volgende woorden uit het gesprek:

1. delen –
2. aankomen (in gewicht) –
3. kort en dik –
4. ervaringen –
5. lichaamsbeweging –
6. uit elkaar gaan –
7. achterwege laten, laten gaan –
8. trainingsschema –
9. moeilijk –
10. overslaan –
11. eigendunk, trots –
12. passen –
13. stimulans –
14. bereiken –

15.	streefgewicht	–
16.	resultaten	–
17.	aanmoediging	–
18.	toegewijd/overtuigd zijn	–
19.	zelfbeeld	–
20.	(zelf)vertrouwen	–

6.3 Speaking and research

Advice on health and safety by the telephone

Find out which health and [safety rules] apply in your job. Write down a number of things that are important. After that you work in pairs and [rehearse] a roleplay in which one person asks for advice per telephone and the other gives information. Below there are sentences that you could use.
Examples for topics to discuss are:
– safety procedures;
– fire exits;
– smoking;
– [use] and [availability] of [protective clothing];
– accidents in the work place;
– use of machines.

ON THE PHONE

You can introduce yourself by saying:
– This is Carol Lynley speaking.
– Hello, this is Carol Lynley.

You can ask for something or someone by saying:
– Could I speak to your health and safety [officer], please?
– I'd like to speak to Ms Glenns, please.
– I'd like him to call me back.
– Could you put me through to the information desk, please?
– Could I speak to someone who…

Examples of questions to ask:
– How do I report accidents?
– How do I know if I need [protective clothing]?
– Where can I go for [health checks]?
– What are my safety [responsibilities] on the job?
– How can I protect my [back]?
– How can I protect my staff against aggressive clients?
– What can I do if I feel no longer safe?
– What can I do if the care and safety of [service users] is no longer [adequate]?
Examples of problems are:
– I'm sorry, I don't understand. Could you [repeat] that, please?
– I'm sorry, I can't hear you very well. Could you [speak up] a little, please?
– I've tried to get through several times but it's always [engaged].
– Could you [spell] that, please?

6.4
Grammar: Adjectives and Adverbs

Een *adjective* of bijvoeglijk naamwoord is een woord dat iets zegt over een zelfstandig naamwoord of een zelfstandig voornaamwoord.

| De uitslag was *slecht*. | – | The result was *bad*. |
| Zij is een *serieus* iemand. | – | She is a *serious* person. |

Bijvoeglijke naamwoorden worden ook gebruikt na werkwoorden van zintuiglijke waarneming.

| Ik voel me *goed*. | – | I'm feeling *fine*. |
| Het eten ruikt *lekker*. | – | The food smells *good*. |

Een *adverb* of bijwoord is een woord of groep woorden die een werkwoord beschrijven of iets aan de betekenis van een werkwoord, een bijvoeglijk naamwoord, een ander bijwoord of een hele zin toevoegen.

Ze bereidde het overleg *nauwkeurig* voor.	–	She *carefully* prepared the meeting.
Zijn tanden waren *erg* slecht.	–	His teeth were *very* bad.
Het gebeurde *verrassend* snel.	–	It happened *surprisingly* quickly.
Natuurlijk, komt de dokter vandaag langs.	–	*Naturally*, the doctor will see you today.

Een bijwoord wordt meestal gevormd door het **bijvoeglijk naamwoord+ -ly**.

| Echt: | real | – | **really** |
| Slecht: | bad | – | **badly** |

Let op!
Uitzondering: het bijwoord van *good* is *well*.

| Zij is een goede adviseur. | – | She is a **good** counsellor. |
| Zij helpt goed | – | She helps **well**. |

Exercise

Vul het goede woord in.
1 The driver was _____ injured. (*serious / seriously*)
2 The driver had _____ injuries. (*serious / seriously*)

3 She hurt herself _____ . (bad / badly)
4 He felt very _____ . (bad / badly)
5 I am not very _____ in English. (good / well)
6 The child behaved _____ . (good / well)
7 This treatment is very _____ . (good / well)
8 Bones are shaped _____ .(different / differently)
9 The students work _____ .They never stop! (continuous / continuously)
10 I cooked this meal _____ for you. (special / specially)

6.5 Research and Writing

Sexual health

First read the information.

KEY FACTS ON SEXUAL HEALTH

- Research [suggests] that sexual [risktaking behaviour] is [increasing] [across] the [population].
- In Western Europe by the end of June 2005 a total of 230,117 HIV infections had been reported in 21 countries. This [understates] the true figure because not all [prevalent] HIV infections have been diagnosed or [reported]. This is partly because many people do not know that they are infected. Of the 23,246 people with newly diagnosed HIV that the West reported in 2004:
- Heterosexual contact has been the most [frequent] [transmission mode] in the West since 1999. It is [responsible] for the largest proportion of diagnosed HIV infections in every country except Germany, Denmark, Greece and the Netherlands, in which men who have sex with men form the largest transmission group. Heterosexual transmission [predominates] even in Portugal, which has a [severe] HIV epidemic [among] [injecting drug users].
- [Chlamydia] is the most [common] [sexually transmitted] infection (STI) and [affects] an [estimated] one in ten sexually active young women. Infections reported in sexual health clinics increased by 9% to over 89,000 in 2003. If left [untreated] it can lead to [pelvic inflammatory] disease, [ectopic pregnancy] and [infertility].
- Other STIs are also increasing. In 2003, cases of [genital warts] increased by 2% to 70,883 and [syphilis] increased by 28% to 1,575.
- [Delays] in [access] to diagnoses and treatment lead to more people being infected with STIs.
- Women, young people, [gay] men, black and [ethnic minority] groups are [disproportionately] [affected] by [poor sexual health].

Exercise

Write a short [essay] on any of the subjects relating to sexual health [mentioned] in the text. Use the internet to do extra research on the subject.
- If you write about any of diseases you should [include]:
- If you write about your sexual health you should include:
- If you write about why some people are more [affected] by poor sexual health than others you should include:
- [Examples] of and [figures] on this group of people;

– the reason for this situation;
– how you feel about it;
– a solution or ideas to change it.

6.6
Reading and research

Anatomy

Zoek Engelstalige informatie op over het menselijk lichaam. Zet daarna de woorden op de juiste plek.

The human body.

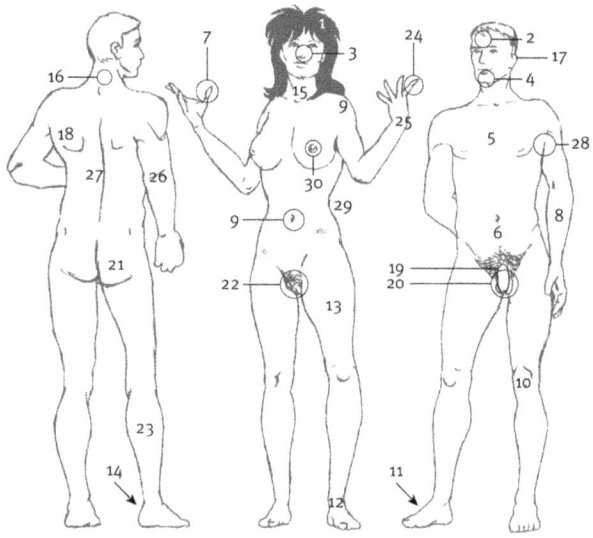

1.
2.
3.
4.
5.
6.
7.
8.
9.
10.
11.
12.
13.
14.
15.

16.
17.
18.
19.
20.
21.
22.
23.
24.
25.
26.
27.
28.
29.
30.

6.7 Grammar

The Plural

In het Engels vorm je *The Plural* (het meervoud) met een **-s**.
Woorden die eindigen op een *s-klank* krijgen **-es**.
Woorden die eindigen op een *medeklinker + y* krijgen **-ies** en de -y valt weg.

bus	–	buses
baby	–	babies

Let op!

potato	–	potatoes
tomato	–	tomatoes

Let op!
In het Engels wordt het meervoud nooit gevormd door **s**.
Er is echter een aantal uitzonderingen.

1. Verandering van medeklinkers:

calf	–	calves (*kuit*)
life	–	lives
self	–	selves
wife	–	wives

2. Verandering van klinkers:

man	–	men
woman	–	women
tooth	–	teeth (*tand*)
foot	–	feet

3. Toevoeging van -en:

child – children
ox – oxen

4. Woorden die gelijk blijven:
Chinese
means (*middelen*)
species (*soorten*)

5. Woorden die alleen enkelvoud hebben:
abuse (misbruik)
progress (vooruitgang)
information

6. Woorden die alleen meervoud hebben:
contents (inhoud)
scissors (schaar)
glasses (bril)

Exercise

Vertaal de woorden die tussen haakjes staan.
1 The _____ are playing outside. (kinderen)
2 The _____ are talking about their _____. (mannen, tanden)
3 What _____ do we have to finish this job? (middelen)
4 The _____ were under the _____. (schaar, kranten)
5 They say _____ have nine _____. (katten, levens)
6 _____ are very healthy. (aardappelen)
7 Do you know the _____ of these _____? (inhoud, dozen)
8 The man had four _____! (echtgenotes)
9 I have been up on my _____ all day. (voeten)
10 She has been to many different _____. (landen)

6.8 Idioms

Exercise

Zoek eerst de woorden op die je niet kent. Probeer hierna met de woorden een correcte Engelse zin te maken.
1. [committee] – present – [sanitary measures]

2. education – sex – condoms

3. health – [condition] – body

4. [scheme] – mothers – [nutrition]

5. [pollution] – protect – [environment]

6. vitamins – healthy

7. alcoholic – [addicted] – alcohol

8. smoking – risk – lung cancer

9. [fresh] – water – drinking

10. [poison] – [absorbed] – [skin]

6.9 Writing and Conversation

Healthy way of life

Try to find out how healthy you are by filling in the [health chart]. You can use the health questions below.

My health chart

Good points	Bad points	Things I have to change	How to change

Health questions:
- How healthy is my diet? Think about vitamins, fruit, vegetables, dairy products, fat, liquids, minerals, fibre.
- What about my level of [physical exercise]?
- How is my personal hygiene?
- How is my sexual hygiene?
- Do I drink alcohol?
- Do I smoke?
- What do I do to [improve] my health?

- How is my [weight]?
- How is my [blood pressure]?
- How healthy is my ([future]) work environment?

After you have completed the chart, work in pairs and interview each other to find out how healthy the other person is.
- Who is the healthiest?
- Can you give the other person advice on how to change things?

6.10 Reading

Good mental health is something you do.

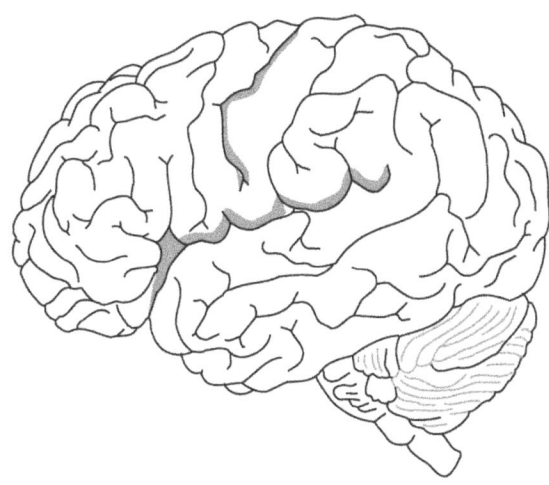

[State of mind]: What keeps people [mentally] well?

Good mental health isn't something you have but something you do. To be mentally healthy you must value and accept yourself. This means that:
You care about and for yourself. You love yourself, not hate yourself. You look after your physical health.
Eat well, sleep well, exercise and [enjoy] yourself.
You see yourself as being a [valuable] person in your own right. You don't have to earn the right to [exist]. You exist, so you have the right to exist.
You [judge] yourself on [reasonable] standards. You don't set yourself [impossible] [goals], such as 'I have to be perfect in everything I do', and then [punish] yourself when you don't [reach] those goals.

If you don't value and accept yourself, then you will always be [frightened] that other people will [reject] you. To prevent people seeing how unacceptable you are, you keep them at a [distance], and so you are always frightened and [lonely]. If you value yourself, then you don't expect people to reject you. You aren't frightened of other people. You can be open and so you enjoy good relationships. If you value and accept yourself, then you are able to relax and enjoy yourself without feeling [guilty]. When you face a crisis you know that, [no matter how] difficult the situation is, you will [manage]. How we see ourselves is [central] to every [decision] we make. People who value and accept themselves [cope] with life.

Exercise

How is your state of mind?

Zoek uit de onderste rij **twee** Engelse vertalingen voor de volgende Nederlandse stemmingen:

1. verdrietig –
2. blij –
3. teruggetrokken –
4. somber –
5. boos –
6. geërgerd –
7. depressief –
8. geïrriteerd –
9. bang –
10. overstuur –

happy, sad, angry, mournful, cheerful, withdrawn, retired, shaken, gloomy, dark, irritated, mad, annoyed, agitated, depressed, low, edgy, afraid, scared, upset

Appendix A

Irregular verbs (onregelmatige werkwoorden)

Hele werkwoord	Verleden tijd	Voltooid deelwoord	Vertaling
Base	Past tense	-ed participle	translation
be	was, were	been	zijn
become	became	become	worden
begin	began	begun	beginnen
bleed	bled	bled	bloeden
break	broke	broken	breken
bring	brought	brought	brengen
buy	bought	bought	kopen
catch	caught	caught	vangen
choose	chose	chosen	kiezen
come	came	come	komen
cut	cut	cut	snijden
do	did	done	doen
drink	drank	drunk	drinken
drive	drove	driven	rijden
eat	ate	eaten	eten
fall	fell	fallen	vallen
feed	fed	fed	(z.) voeden
feel	felt	felt	(z.) voelen
find	found	found	vinden
fly	flew	flown	vliegen
forget	forgot	forgotten	vergeten
freeze	froze	frozen	(be)vriezen
get	got	got	krijgen
give	gave	given	geven
go	went	gone	gaan
grow	grew	grown	groeien
have	had	had	hebben
hear	heard	heard	horen
hurt	hurt	hurt	bezeren, pijn doen
keep	kept	kept	houden
know	knew	known	weten

Hele werkwoord Base	Verleden tijd Past tense	Voltooid deelwoord -ed participle	Vertaling translation
leave	left	left	(ver)laten
lose	lost	lost	verliezen
make	made	made	maken
mean	meant	meant	bedoelen
meet	met	met	ontmoeten
pay	paid	paid	betalen
put	put	put	leggen, zetten
read	read	read	lezen
ring	rang	rung	bellen
rise	rose	risen	opstaan, stijgen
run	ran	run	hardlopen
say	said	said	zeggen
see	saw	seen	zien
sell	sold	sold	verkopen
send	sent	sent	zenden, sturen
show	showed	shown	laten zien
sit	sat	sat	zitten
sleep	slept	slept	slapen
speak	spoke	spoken	spreken
spend	spent	spent	uitgeven, doorbrengen
stand	stood	stood	staan
steal	stole	stolen	stelen
sweep	swept	swept	vegen
swim	swam	swum	zwemmen
take	took	taken	nemen
teach	taught	taught	leren, onderwijzen
tell	told	told	vertellen, zeggen
think	thought	thought	denken
understand	understood	understood	begrijpen
weep	wept	wept	huilen
win	won	won	winnen
write	wrote	written	schrijven

Appendix B

Vocabulary English – Dutch

Deze woorden staan tussen [ ] in de tekst. De vertaling van de woorden heeft betrekking op de bijbehorende tekst.

ability	vermogen
abroad	in het buitenland
absorb (to)	opnemen
abuse	misbruik
access	toegang
accident	ongeluk
accommodation	onderdak, woning
accomplish (to)	bereiken
according to	volgens
accountable	verantwoordelijk
accountability	aansprakelijkheid
achieve (to)	bereiken
achievement	prestatie
acids	zuren
actually	echt, eigenlijk
acquaintances	kennissen
acquire (to)	opdoen van ziekte
across	door/in heel
add (to)	toevoegen
addicted	verslaafd
adequate	voldoende
adhere (to)	zich houden aan
adult	volwassene
advert	advertentie
advertise (to)	adverteren
advertisement	advertentie
affairs	zaken, kwesties
affect (to)	beïnvloeden
age	leeftijd
agitated	geïrriteerd
agree with (to)	eens zijn met

agreement	verdrag
aim	doel(stelling)
aimed at	gericht op
affairs	zaken, kwesties
agreement	verdrag
alarm clock	wekker
allegation	beschuldiging
allowance	tegoed
allowed (to be) (to)	mogen, toestemming hebben
already	al
although	hoewel
amazing	verbazingwekkend
amino acids	aminozuren
among	onder
amount	hoeveelheid
announce (to)	aankondigen
annoyance	irritatie
anxieties	punten van zorg
apathetic	onverschillig
apparently	blijkbaar
appeal (to)	aantrekken, leuk vinden
appear (to)	lijken
applaud (to)	toejuichen
applicant	sollicitant
apply (to)	solliciteren
appointment	afspraak
arrange (to)	regelen
arrangement	regeling
assess	beoordelen
assessment	beoordeling, evaluatie
assume (to)	aannemen
at once	tegelijk
at one time	ooit
at short notice	snel, zonder waarschuwing
attach (to)	verbonden
attitude	houding
auctions	veilingen
audience	publiek
available	beschikbaar
availability	beschikbaarheid
(on) average	in het algemeen
avoid (to)	vermijden
awareness	bewustzijn
back	rug

background	achtergrond
bad behaviour	slecht gedrag
bad temper	slecht humeur
balance (to)	in evenwicht brengen
balanced	evenwichtig
bandage	verband
bank account	bankrekening
bank holiday	officiële feestdag op een werkdag
bank statement	afschrijving
be all and the end all	het enige wat telt
become (to)	worden
behave (to)	gedragen
behaviour	gedrag
beliefs	overtuigingen
belongings	bezittingen
benefit (to)	voordeel hebben van
benefit from (to)	iets hebben van
benefits	uitkering
betray (to)	bedriegen, misbruiken
bill (to)	in rekening brengen
block of flats	flatgebouw
blood pressure	bloeddruk
body language	lichaamstaal
body tissues	lichaamsweefsels
body weight	lichaamsgewicht
bored (to be)	zich vervelen
boring	saai
borrow (to)	lenen
boss around (to)	de baas spelen over
breach (to)	overtreden
break	pauze, vrije dag
brighter	fleuriger
budget (to)	budgetteren
bulk	massa, volume
bullied	geïntimideerd, gepest
bully (to)	intimideren, pesten
burn (down) (to)	afbranden
busy	druk
call	telefoongesprek
call (to)	opbellen
call for	oproep tot
call minutes	belminuten
call (to) names	uitschelden
campaign	campagne

canteen food	voedsel in de kantine
capacity	talent, vaardigheid / vermogen
carbohydrates	koolhydraten
care	zorg
care assistant	helpende
career goals	loopbaandoelen
career test	beroepskeuzetest
career/work history	werkervaring
care for the elderly	ouderenzorg
careful	voorzichtig
carer	(mantel)zorger
care worker	hulpverlener
carry forward (to)	meenemen
case study	gevalsanalyse
cashflow	kasstroom
central	belangrijk
certain	bepaald
change (to)	wisselen, verschonen
charge (to)	in rekening brengen
(in) charge of	leiding hebben over
chart	lijst, overzicht
cheap	goedkoop
cheerful	vrolijk
chemicals	chemische stoffen
child welfare office	bureau voor kinderbescherming
children's home	kindertehuis
Chlamydia	Chlamydia (bacterie)
choice	keuze
chore	klusje
circumstances	omstandigheden
citizenship	burgerschap
clearly	duidelijk
close	hecht, nauw
code of conduct	gedragscode
code of Practice	gedragscode
cohesion	samenhang
colleagues	collega's
collect (to)	ophalen
college	hoge school (hbo)
come across (to)	tegenkomen
comment (to)	commentaar geven
commissioner	commissaris
commitment	overtuiging, betrokkenheid
committee	commissie

common	veel voorkomend
common sense	gezond verstand
community	extramuraal, wijk
community centre	buurt/wijkcentrum
Communist rule	Communistische regering
compared to	vergeleken met
comparisons	vergelijkingen
complain (to)	klagen
complaint	klacht
complete (to)	uitvoeren
comprise (to)	opgebouwd zijn uit
concern (to)	betreffen
condition	aandoening, toestand
Conduct Committee	Gedragscommissie
confident	vol zelfvertrouwen
confidential information	vertrouwelijke informatie
confused	verward
connect (to)	verbonden
consent	toestemming
consider to	overwegen
considered	doordacht
constant	voortdurend
construction	opbouw
consumer	klant, consument
contain (to)	bevatten
contribute to (to)	bijdragen aan
controlled deep breathing	ademhalingstechniek
conversation	gesprek
cope (to)	kunnen omgaan met
correct (to)	verbeteren
correspondence	briefwisseling
Council	raad
counsellor	psycho-sociaal hulpverlener
count	telling
count (to)	(mee)tellen
country (in the)	op het platteland
cover (to)	gaan over, beslaan
cover up (to)	bedekken
coverage	dekking
co-worker	directe collega
crammed into	op elkaar gepropt
creep back on (to)	langzaam terugkomen
creep up (to)	besluipen
critisize (to)	kritiek hebben op

curl up (to)	oprollen tot
customer	klant, cliënt
cut off (to)	stoppen, onderbreken
daily	dagelijks
daily living activities	activiteiten dagelijkse leven
damaged	beschadigd
days off	vrije dagen
deal with (to)	bezighouden / omgaan met
debt	schuld
decide (to)	beslissen
decision	beslissing
decision making	besluitvorming
deck	dek (van een boot)
dedicate (to)	wijden aan
delay	vertraging
deliver (to)	bieden aan
delivery	bezorging
demand (to)	eisen
dentist	tandarts
deny (to)	ontkennen
department	afdeling
depend on (to)	afhangen van
design (to)	ontwerpen
despite	ondanks
destress (to)	ontstressen
detailed	gedetailleerd
details	informatie
deteriorate (to)	achteruitgaan
determine (to)	vastleggen
determination	vastbeslotenheid
develop (to)	ontwikkelen
development	ontwikkeling
diabetes	suikerziekte
diary	agenda, logboek
difference	verschil
different	verschillend(e)
differently	anders
difficulties	problemen
disabled	gehandicapt
disability	handicap
discipline (to)	straffen
disease	ziekte
dishonesty	oneerlijkheid
dismiss (to)	ontslaan

disproportionately	buiten proportie (te hoog/laag)
distance	afstand
diversity	gevarieerdheid
dress (to)	aankleden
dress code	kledingvoorschrift
Dutch	Nederlanders
duty of care	zorgplicht
each	elk
earn (to)	verdienen
ectopic pregnancy	buitenbaarmoederlijke zwangerschap
economic interest	economisch belang
education	onderwijs
educational setting	opleidingsplek
either	ook niet
elder(ly)	oudere
elect (to)	kiezen
eligible (to be)	in aanmerking komen voor
emergency	noodgeval
employ (to)	werk bieden aan
employee	werknemer
employer	werkgever
employment	werkgelegenheid
empower (to)	in staat stellen
(to) enable	in staat stellen
encourage (to)	aanmoedigen
engaged (to be)	bezet zijn (telefoon)
engaged in (to be)	bezig zijn met
enjoy (to)	leuk vinden, bezitten
ensure (to)	zeker stellen van
environment	omgeving, milieu
equal	hetzelfde, evenveel
equal opportunities	gelijke rechten
equipment	hulpmiddel
essay	opstel, essay
essential	noodzakelijk
especially	vooral
establish	winnen, vestigen
estate	(woon)wijk
estimated	geschat aantal
estimation	schatting
ethical value	ethische (meer)waarde
ethnic minority	etnische minderheid
EU	Europese Unie
evaluation	evaluatiegesprek

evidence	bewijsmateriaal
examples	voorbeelden
excess	te veel
exchanges	uitwisselingen
exchange students	uitwisselingsstudenten
exercise	lichaamsbeweging
exercise of	uitoefening van
exist (to)	bestaan
exit	uitgang
expect (to)	verwachten
expenditure	uitgaven
expensive	duur
experience (to)	ervaren
expertise	kennis, deskundigheid
explain (to)	uitleggen
expulsion	van school afsturen
extend (to)	uitbreiden
face (to)	onder ogen zien
factual	feitelijk
fail (to)	zakken, mislukken
fair	eerlijk
fairly	nogal
fall below (to)	niet voldoen aan
fall into debt (to)	schulden krijgen
false	niet waar
false claim	valse beschuldiging
farming	landbouw
fault (to be at)	fout zijn
fed up (to be)	beu zijn
fee	kosten
fellow students	medestudenten
fibres	vezels
figures	bedragen, getallen
file (to)	indienen
fill in (to)	invullen
fit in (to)	passen bij
first aid	eerste hulp
flee (to)	vluchten
focus on (to)	zich richten op
focus of attention	nadruk
for instance	bijvoorbeeld
formidable	enorm
foster placements	opvangplaatsen
frail	kwetsbaar

freedom of expression	vrijheid van meningsuiting
frequent	vaak voorkomend
fresh	vers
frightened	bang
functional relation	functionele (werk)relatie
fundamental	belangrijk, hoofd-
fundamental values	basiswaarden
future	toekomstig
gay	homoseksueel
gender	geslacht
general	algemeen
generate (to)	opwekken
genital warts	wratten in geslachtsstreek
gently	rustig, aardig
genuine	oprecht
get (to) into trouble	in de problemen raken
gift	cadeau
glue	lijm
goal	doel(stelling)
government	regering
GP (general practitioner)	huisarts
grab rail	handsteun, -greep
gradually	geleidelijk
grant (to)	toestaan
grasp	grip
grateful	dankbaar
grave	ernstig
growth spurt	groeispurt
GSCC	Algemene Raad Maatschappelijk Werk
guarantee	garantie
guaranteed income	vast inkomen
guilty	schuldig
habit	gewoonte
hairdresser	kapper
handle (to)	omgaan met
handset	telefoon
harm (to)	schade toebrengen aan
hazard	gevaar
head of state	staatshoofd
health care	gezondheidszorg
health centre	gezondheidscentrum
health chart	gezondheidstabel
health checks	gezondheidsonderzoek
health education	gezondheidsvoorlichting

health workers	gezondheidswerkers
hidden	verstopt
hint	aanwijzing
hold	scheepsruim
homeless person	dakloze
homogeneous	gelijksoortig
horrible	afschuwelijk
host	veel
hostel	tehuis, opvang
housing problems	huisvestingsproblemen
humiliate (to)	vernederen
hurt (to get)	gewond raken
identify (to)	bekendmaken, vaststellen
ideology	ideologie, gedachtenstelsel
ignore (to)	negeren, ontkennen
ignorant	onwetend, dom
ill	ziek
illness	ziekte
imagine (to)	inbeelden
immediately	onmiddellijk
impartial	onpartijdig
imply (to)	inhouden
important	belangrijk
impossible	onmogelijk
impression	indruk
improve (to)	verbeteren
in accordance with	in overeenstemming met
inappropriate	ongepaste
incident	voorval
include (to)	omvatten
income	inkomsten
incompetent	ondeskundig
incompetence	ondeskundigheid
increase (to)	verhogen
increasingly	toenemend
in debt (to be in)	schulden hebben
independence	onafhankelijkheid
independent	onafhankelijk
industry	industrie
infertility	onvruchtbaarheid
influence (to)	beïnvloeden
in full	voluit
inhale (to)	inademen
injecting drug users	intraveneuze drugsgebruikers

APPENDIX B

injured	gewond
insist (to)	aandringen
instill (to)	bijbrengen
interests	belangen
interest charges	berekende rente
interest group	belangengroep/-vereniging
introduce (to)	voorstellen
involve (to)	betrekken
issues	kwestie, probleem
items	voorwerpen
join (to)	lid worden van
journey	reis, trip
judge (to)	beoordelen
judgement	oordeel
juggle (to)	combineren, goochelen
keep (to)	bewaren
key	sleutel, toegang
kind	aardig
knowledge	kennis
lack of	ontbreken van
language	taal
lay down (to)	voorschrijven
letter of application	sollicitatiebrief
lads	jongens
launch (to)	van start laten gaan
launch	lancering, start
law	wet
leaflet	folder
legal duty	wettelijke plicht
legally	wettelijk
legislation	wetgeving
level	niveau
life experience	levenservaring
lies and rumours	leugens en roddels
likely	waarschijnlijk
likely (to be to)	neiging hebben tot
limited	beperkt
limits	grenzen
limp	mank
live off (to)	leven van
local authority	lokale overheid
look after (to)	zorgen voor
look ahead (to)	vooruitkijken
look for (to)	zoeken

loan	lening
lonely	alleen
loudly	luid, heel hard
lower (to)	verlagen
luckily	gelukkig
lunch break	lunchpauze
main	belangrijk, hoofd-
maintain (to)	behouden
make ends meet (to)	eindjes aan elkaar knopen
manage (to)	aankunnen, sturen
managed by (to be)	bestuurd worden door
map	plattegrond
marital status	burgerlijke staat (on/gehuwd enz.)
maternity leave	zwangerschapsverlof
matter	zaak
matter (to)	er toe doen
maximize	zo groot mogelijk maken
mean (to)	betekenen
mechanic	monteur
meet (to)	voldoen aan, elkaar ontmoeten
member	lid
mental health nurse	psychatrieverpleegkundige
mental nursing	psychiatrieverpleging
mentally	geestelijk, psychisch
mention (to)	noemen
mess up (to)	er een puinhoop van maken
method of payment	betalingswijze
midwifery	voor de verloskundigen
misconduct	wangedrag
misleading	misleidend
mongrel	bastaard
mount up (to)	meer worden
movement	beweging, organisatie
muscles	spieren
muscle tension	spierspanning
mutual	wederzijds
mutual understanding	wederzijds begrip
navy	marine
necessary	nodig
necklace	ketting
need	behoefte
neglect	verwaarlozing
neighbours	buren
night shift	nachtdienst

no matter how	hoe dan ook
non-violent	geweldloos
note down (to)	opschrijven
not simply	niet alleen
nowadays	tegenwoordig
number	aantal
nurse	verpleegkundige
nursing home	verpleeghuis
nursing unit	verpleegafdeling
nutrition	voeding
obese	dik, overgewicht
obtain consent	toestemming krijgen
obvious	duidelijk
occasional	af en toe
occupational safety	veiligheid op het werk
of course	natuurlijk
offer (to)	aanbieden
officer	functionaris, agent
often	vaak
omission	weglating
ongoing	doorgaand
operate (to)	optreden
opportunity	mogelijkheid
oppose (to)	verzetten tegen
opposite	tegenovergestelde
out of date	gedateerd, achterhaald
overdo (to)	te veel vergen
overdrafts	bankschulden
overhear	meeluisteren
overload (to)	overladen
overtime	overwerk
owe (to)	schuldig zijn
owner	eigenaar
oxygen	zuurstof
package	pakket
paediatric ward	kinderafdeling
pairs	tweetallen
pass (to)	slagen
parental leave	ouderschapsverlof
parliament	parlement, volksvertegenwoordiging
parliamentary adviser	palementair adviseur
part and parcel	onmisbaar onderdeel van
participants	deelnemers
participate (to)	doen aan

partnership	samenwerking
pass (to)	slagen voor examen
peak times	piektijden
pelvic inflammation	bekkenonsteking
performance	uitvoering, prestatie
performance interview	functioneringsgesprek
perspective	kijk op
physical exercise	lichaamsbeweging
physical or mental	lichamelijk of geestelijk
pick (to) on	vitten, afgeven op
pin (to)	vastklemmen
play garden	speeltuin
plea (to)	pleiten
pocket money	zakgeld
pointer	tip
poison	vergif
policies	beleid
policy maker	beleidsmaker
policies and procedures	beleid en methodes
polite	beleefd
pollution	vervuiling
poor health	slechte gezondheid
poor sexual health	slechte seksuele gezondheid
population	bevolking
position	houding
power	macht
practice	praktijk, werk
practice (to)	oefenen
predominate (to)	overheersen
prejudice	vooroordeel
premium rate	duurste tarief
prepare (to)	voorbereiden
prepared	voorbereid
press	media (tv, kranten)
pressure	druk
pressure group	belangenvereniging
prevalent	voorkomend
prevent (to)	voorkomen
primarly task	eerste taak
prime minister	minister president, premier
prior	voorafgaand
private care	particuliere zorg
probably	waarschijnlijk
profession	beroepsgroep

professional	beroepskracht
professional attitude	beroepshouding
prominent	belangrijk
promising	veelbelovend
promote (to)	stimuleren
probably	waarschijnlijk
properly	goed, juist
protect (to)	beschermen
protection	bescherming
protective clothing	beschermende kleding
proteins	eiwitten
prove (to)	bewijzen
provide (to)	bieden (aan), leveren
provision	het voorzien
psychological	psychisch
public	voor iedereen
public services	overheidsdiensten
punish (to)	straffen
pupils	studenten
purpose	doel
put forward (to)	naar voren brengen
put up with (to)	accepteren
qualification	diploma
qualified	gediplomeerd
quality (of life)	kwaliteit (van leven), leefbaarheid
quietly	stilletjes
quite right	helemaal juist
rape (to)	verkrachten
rate	tarief
reach (to)	bereiken
readable	leesbaar
reasonable	redelijk
recognise (to)	herkennen, onderkennen
recommend (to)	aanbevelen
records	aantekeningen, gegevens
recover (to)	herstellen
redecorate (to)	opknappen, schilderen
refer (to)	verwijzen naar
referenda	stemronde
refugee centre	vluchtelingencentrum
refuse (to)	weigeren
regardless	om het even
registered	gediplomeerd
registered practitioner	ingeschreven beroepsbeoefenaar

regularly	regelmatig
rehearse (to)	oefenen
reject (to)	afwijzen
reliance	vertrouwen
remain (to)	blijven
reminder	geheugensteuntje
remove (to)	verwijderen
repeat (to)	herhalen
report	rapport
report (to)	aangeven (bij de politie), melden
request	verzoek
require (to)	vereisen
reside (to)	wonen
resident	bewoner
residential home	verzorgingshuis
resolution	oplossen van
resolve (to)	oplossen
resource	bron
respond to (to)	reageren op
response	reactie
responsible	verantwoordelijk
responsibilities	verantwoordelijkheden
responsive to (to be)	ontvankelijk voor
restrain (to)	in bedwang houden
review (to)	heroverwegen
rights and duties	rechten en plichten
risky	risicovol
risktaking behaviour	risicogedrag
roughage	ruwe vezels
rudeness	lompheid, onbeleefdheid
rule of law	rechtsorde
run (to)	organiseren
safety	veiligheid
safety issues	veiligheidskwesties
safety measures	veiligheidsmaatregelen
safety rules	veiligheidsregels
sales assistant	verkoopmedewerkster
sanitary measures	gezondheidsmaatregelen
scary	eng
schedules	(tijd)schema's
scheme	programma, plan
salary	salaris
seek (to)	proberen, streven
sell (to)	verkopen

senior	ouder, meer ervaren
sensible	verstandig
separately	apart
serious	ernstig
seriously	echt waar
services	diensten
service users	cliënten
services sector	dienstensector
setting	omgeving
set format	één manier
set out (to)	opstellen, beschrijven
severe	ernstig
sexually transmitted	seksueel overgedragen
shame (what a)	wat jammer
sheets	formulieren
shin	scheenbeen
side (to)	partij kiezen voor
similarity	overeenkomst
single	eenmalig
skill	vaardigheid
skin	huid
skin condition	huidaandoening
Social Affairs	Sociale Zaken
social care services	sociale voorzieningen
social worker	maatschappelijk werker
solely	alleen
solution	oplossing
solve (to)	oplossen
sore	pijnlijk
spare time activities	hobbies
speak up (to)	harder praten
speech	toespraak
spell (to)	spellen
spend (to)	doorbrengen, geld uitgeven
spending	uitgaven
spokeswoman	woordvoerdster
square	plein
state of mind	gemoedstoestand
statistics	cijfers van onderzoek
stock	voorraad
store manager	directeur van de winkel
straight away	meteen
strain	spanning
strengthen (to)	versterken

strengths	sterke kanten
stretch (to)	oprekken
strict	streng
strive (to)	streven naar
struck (to)	opvallen
struggle (to)	worstelen
students' council	studentenraad
stuff like that	dat soort dingen
subject	onderwerp
subscriber	ondertekenaars, abonnees
subscription	abonnement
substances	stoffen
suffer from (to)	lijden aan
suggest (to)	(lijkt te)wijzen op
suit (to)	passen bij
summary	samenvatting
support	ondersteuning
suppose (to)	veronderstellen
sure (to be)	er zeker van zijn
syphilis	syfilis (geslachtsziekte)
tackle (to)	aanpakken, oplossen
tailor	kleermaker
tailored	op maat gemaakt
tariff	tarief
tease (to)	plagen
teenager	tiener
tend to (to)	neiging hebben tot
telly	tv
territorial waters	driemijlszone (grens)
theft	diefstal
thorough	grondig
threat	dreiging
tissues	weefsels
topic	onderwerp
train (to)	opgeleid worden voor
traineeships	stages
transfer (to)	overplaatsen
transmission mode	manier van overbrengen
travel (to)	reizen
treat (to)	verwennen
true	waar
trust	vertrouwen
trustworthy	betrouwbaar
turn against (to)	tegen iemand richten

twist (to)	verdraaien
ultimately	uiteindelijk
underpin (to)	onderbouwen
understate (to)	te laag opgeven
undertake (to)	ondernemen, uitvoeren
unemployment figures	werkloosheidscijfers
unfair	oneerlijk
unfortunately	helaas
union	vakbond
unite (to)	verenigen, samen brengen
Universal Declaration	Universele Verklaring
unlawful	onwettig
unnecessary	onnodig
unpleasantness	onplezierig gedrag
unreasonable	onredelijk
unreasonable demands	onredelijke eisen
unruly	onhandelbaar
untreated	onbehandeld
unused	ongebruikt
up front	van tevoren
uphold (to)	in stand houden
usage	gebruik
usage pattern	gebruikerspatroon
usually	meestal
unwise	onverstandig
use	gebruik
useful	nuttig
usually	meestal
vague	vaag
valuable	waardevol
vandalism	vandalisme, vernielzucht
vary (to)	variëren, afwisselen
victim	slachtoffer
view	mening
violence	geweld
violent	gewelddadig
visualisation	visualisatie, zich voorstellen
voice	stem
vote (to)	stemmen
voting age	leeftijd waarop iemand mag stemmen
voucher	tegoedbon
vulnerable	kwetsbaar
waste disposal fee	verwijderingsbijdrage

walking frame	looprekje
wander off (to)	weglopen
ward	afdeling
warning signs	waarschuwingssignalen
waste products	afvalproducten, ontlasting
watch closely (to)	in de gaten houden
weight	gewicht
welfare	welzijn
welfare officer	welzijnswerker
well off (to be)	rijk zijn
wellbeing	welzijn
went down (to go down)	minder worden
wheelchair	rolstoel
whether	of
whereabouts	verblijfplaats
while	terwijl
whilst	terwijl
white coffee	koffie met melk
WHO	Wereldgezondheidsorganisatie
Witness	getuigen
workforce	beroepsbevolking
working order	functionerend
workplace steward	vakbondsvertegenwoordiger
worry (to)	zorgen maken over
worse	slecht(er)
wrong (to go)	fout gaan

Key

Unit 1

1.1 Questions about the text

1. c	6. d	11. c
2. d	7. b	12. a
3. a	8. d	13. d
4. d	9. c	
5. a	10. a	

1.2 How to behave? Idioms

1. code of conduct
2. exaggerated
3. to worry
4. treatment
5. confidential information
6. patient details
7. colleagues
8. dignity
9. policies
10. receive
11. upset (to be)
12. rules
13. protect
14. abuse
15. horror stories
16. cases
17. to know for sure
18. bruises
19. accuses
20. protect

1.3 Research

1. the purpose of the code:
A: to:
- inform the professions of the standard of professional conduct required of them in the exercise of their professional accountability and practice;
- inform the public, other professions and employers of the standard of professional conduct that they can expect of a registered practitioner.

B: to:
- set out the conduct that is expected of social care workers and to inform service users and the public about the standards of conduct they can expect from social care workers.

2. Nurses should:
- respect the patient or client as an individual;
- obtain consent before giving any treatment or care;
- protect confidential information;
- co-operate with others in the team;
- maintain their professional knowledge and competence;
- be trustworthy;
- act to identify and minimise risk to patients and clients.

Social care workers should:
- protect the rights and promote the interests of service users and carers;
- strive to establish and maintain the trust and confidence of service users and carers;
- promote the independence of service users while protecting them as far as possible from danger or harm;
- respect the rights of service users whilst seeking to ensure that their behaviour does not harm themselves or other people;
- uphold public trust and confidence in social care services;
- be accountable for the quality of their work and take responsibility for maintaining and improving their knowledge and skills.

3. Nurses should not:
- disrespect the patient or client as an individual;
- forget to obtain consent before giving any treatment or care;
- give away confidential information;
- refuse to co-operate with others in the team;
- neglect professional knowledge and competence;
- be untrustworthy;
- maximise risk to patients and clients.

Social care workers should not:
- violate the rights or stop to promote the interests of service users and carers;
- stop establishing and maintaining the trust and confidence of service users and carers;
- stop to promote the independence of service users while protecting them as far as possible from danger or harm;
- disrespect the rights of service users whilst seeking to ensure that their behaviour does not harm themselves or other people;
- violate public trust and confidence in social care services;
- stop to be accountable for the quality of their work and take responsibility for maintaining and improving their knowledge and skills.

4. Personal answer.

1.4 Grammar: the Present Tense

1 checks
2 lives
3 come in

KEY 127

4 makes
5 supplies
6 offers
7 brushes
8 cleans
9 likes
10 applies
11 says
12 checks
13 complains
14 have
15 works

1.5 Translation

1 I work mainly with young people.
2 She gives advice and explanation.
3 I come from the Netherlands.
4 I speak English very well.
5 I apply for this post.

1.8 Prepositions

1 with
2 out
3 up
4 after
5 up
6 under
7 with
8 with
9 in
10 by
11 for
12 in
13 up
14 about
15 in
16 with
17 of
18 in
19 for, of
20 with

1.11 Grammar

A THE PRESENT CONTINUOUS TENSE

1 are working
2 am going
3 is waiting
4 am losing

5 are making
6 is raining
7 are talking
8 is reading
9 is learning
10 are waiting

B THE SIMPLE PRESENT TENSE OF THE PRESENT CONTINUOUS TENSE

1 am going
2 speaks
3 does close
4 is raining
5 is getting
6 do work
7 don't eat
8 is learning (2×)
9 drink
10 finishes

Unit 2

2.1 Young people need strong voice

1 b
2 a
3 d
4 a
5 d
6 c
7 d
8 a
9 d
10 c

2.3 Listening Skill 2

1 harassed
2 union member
3 reasons
4 pay
5 compensation
6 discriminated
7 sacked
8 examples
9 student nurse
10 all the way
11 dismissed
12 behaviour
13 joking
14 definitely
15 victim
16 habit

KEY

17 scared
18 It's your call
19 employment rights
20 nothing to lose

2.4 Grammar: The Past Tense

1 calmed
2 ran
3 thought
4 met
5 changed
6 asked
7 worked
8 rang
9 drank
10 took

2.5 Verbs

1 feel
2 are
3 want / need
4 can
5 feel
6 do
7 suffering
8 committed
9 interview
10 pay
11 consult
12 solve
13 do
14 express
15 needs

2.7 Listening Skill 3

1 false
2 true
3 true
4 false
5 true
6 true
7 false
8 true
9 true
10 false

2.8 Translation

1 She protested against his bad behaviour.
2 Greenpeace is a well known interest group.
3 They elected three students.
4 The students decided to vote.
5 He improved the quality of the school.

2.10 A window on Europe: what do you think?

1 inevitable
2 vote
3 involved
4 otherwise
5 it seems
6 knowledge
7 government
8 represent
9 healthily
10 responsibility
11 committee
12 elections
13 diverse
14 European Parliament
15 compared to
16 probably
17 abroad
18 unreasonable views
19 currency
20 laws

Unit 3

3.1 Too many young people are getting hurt at work

1 c
2 a
3 d
4 a
5 d
6 b
7 a
8 c
9 d
10 a

3.2 Performance interview

1 trial period
2 thus far
3 demanding
4 gravity

5 responsibility
6 mess
7 efforts
8 improve
9 insecure
10 condition
11 appointment
12 prepare
13 reports
14 achieves
15 expectations
16 improvement
17 get the hang of it
18 issues
19 enjoy

3.4 Grammar: The Future Tense

1 goed
2 Mike will help
3 Hassan will go
4 goed
5 The new stock will arrive
6 I am going to work
7 goed
8 you will feel
9 goed
10 she is going to make

3.5 Translation

1 Don't be afraid to ask questions.
2 You should get all your medicines from the same pharmacy.
3 If you find it hard to remember you should write it down.
4 Here's a leaflet with some information.
5 We have information available on these appliances.

3.6 Listening Skill 5

1 true
2 false
3 true
4 false
5 true
6 true
7 false
8 false
9 true
10 false

3.8 Grammar: much, many, little, few

1 much
2 many
3 few
4 much
5 little

3.10 Grammar: A or an

1 a
2 a
3 an
4 a
5 an
6 a

Unit 4

4.1 How to choose a mobile service

1 The most important thing is how you expect to use your mobile phone.
2 You want to know whether you have a good signal in these places.
3 Mobile services and prices change so often that any detailed summary or price comparisons would quickly be out of date.
4 By first finding out your needs and usage pattern.
5 Your general usage of the phone.
6 Mobile phone companies' websites, mobile phone shops and Oftel's website.
7 Monthly contract, prepay, pay up front.
8 You have to pay for a minimum contract period of at least 12 months.
9 You pay before making calls, for example with a call voucher.
10 On average, you pay over three times as much, but the difference can be bigger.

Listening skills 6

4.2 I have been robbed!

1 VCR
2 department store
3 to deliver
4 customer's service
5 to inquire
6 to assure
7 claims
8 upset
9 sales manager
10 to look into matters
11 to get in touch
12 to presume
13 refer to
14 to investigate
15 goods

KEY   133

16 to get back to
17 indifference
18 on the part of
19 negligence
20 proof

4.4 Grammar: Questions and Negations

1. The patient is feeling nauseated.
a Is the patient feeling nauseated?
b The patient is not feeling nauseated.

2. The children are hiding underneath the desk.
a Are the children hiding underneath the desk?
b The children are not hiding underneath the desk.

3. The old lady/woman understands what I am talking about.
a Does the old lady/woman understand what I am talking about?
b The old lady/woman does not understand what I am talking about.

4. The doctor walks into the surgery.
a Does the doctor walk into the surgery?
b The doctor does not walk into the surgery.

5. Justin is finishing his paperwork this afternoon.
a Is Justin finishing his paperwork this afternoon?
a Justin is not finishing his paperwork this afternoon.

6. Marjory can tell you how to deal with her.
a Can Marjory tell you how to deal with her?
b Marjory cannot tell you how to deal with her.

7. Ian likes his job/work very much.
a Does Ian like his job/work very much?
b Ian does not like his job/work very much.

8. The girl has lost her parents.
a Has the girl lost her parents?
b The girl has not lost het parents.

9. Older people walk slower than younger people.
a Do older people walk slower than younger people?
b Older people do not walk slower than younger people.

10. Jez has prepared everything for the next meeting.
a Has Jez prepared everything for the next meeting?
b Jez has not prepared everything for the next meeting.

4.5 Translation

1 Where does it hurt?
2 What is the matter?
3 Tell me what has happened.

4 Do you often have a toothache?
5 When were you treated?

4.8 Reading

ARE YOU IN DEBT?

Vraag 4:
emergency – unexpected dangerous situation
straight away – immediately
overdraft – an excess of money spent
to earn – to obtain money for work
to tackle – to deal with
to mount up – to become larger
at short notice – with little warning
fees – money paid for services
to owe – have an obligation to pay
cash flow – amount of money being transferred

4.9 Grammar: Personal and Possessive Pronouns

1 her, hers
2 your, mine
3 he, her, her
4 their
5 She, our
6 his, his
7 your, yours
8 it, my, you, me

4.10 Writing

Numbers

0	nought, zero	–	–	–
1	one	eerste	1st	first
2	two	tweede	2nd	second
3	three	derde	3rd	third
4	four	vierde	4th	fourth
5	five	vijfde	5th	fifth
6	six	zesde	6th	sixth
7	seven	zevende	7th	seventh
8	eight	achtste	8th	eighth
9	nine	negende	9th	ninth
10	ten	tiende	10th	tenth
11	eleven	elfde	11th	eleventh
12	twelve	twaalfde	12th	twelfth
13	thirteen	dertiende	13th	thirteenth

KEY   135

20	twenty	twintigste	20th	twentieth
21	twenty-one	eenentwintig-ste	21st	twenty-first
100	a / one hundred	honderdste	100th	one hundredth
200	two hundred	tweehonderd-ste	200th	two hundredth
1000	a / one thousand	eenduizendste	1,000th	one thousandth
1.000.000	a / one million	eenmiljoenste	1,000,000th	one millionth

Unit 5

5.1 Do we need Citizenship?

1 c
2 a
3 d
4 d
5 a
6 b
7 d
8 a
9 b
10 c

Listening Skills 7

5.2 Private and professional attitude

1 attitude
2 conversation
3 topic of discussion
4 difference
5 day-care centre for children
6 playgroup
7 lose your temper
8 naughty
9 to snap
10 deliberately
11 lose my patience
12 nature
13 intimacy
14 to add
15 stand up for themselves
16 abuse of trust
17 expectations
18 attitude
19 comments
20 unfortunately

5.4 Grammar: The Present Perfect Tense

1 have forgotten
2 has gone
3 have looked
4 has given
5 has made

5.5 Translation

1 We are open from 9 am to 6 pm.
2 You must make an appointment first.
3 You cannot get medicines here.
4 If the complaints are getting worse you should call us back.
5 Who is your landlord?

Listening Skills 8

5.8 Flight from Vietnam

1 flight
2 refugee
3 scared
4 to endanger
5 entry
6 entrance exams
7 background
8 journey
9 dangerous
10 challenge
11 obvious choice
12 to board (boarded)
13 for safety's sake
14 fetal position
15 horrible
16 waves
17 permitted
18 occasionally
19 refugee camp
20 asylum-seekers
21 eligible
22 to enroll
23 screened
24 approved
25 United States

5.9 Grammar: Relative Pronouns

1 who
2 whom
3 that/who

4 which
5 whose

Unit 6

6.1 Food and health

1 eating a balanced diet, taking lots of exercise and avoiding things which damage your body such as smoking
2 damage organs even kill
3 proteins, vitamins, minerals, water, fat, carbohydrates and roughage
4 provide energy
5 acids, amino acids
6 growth and to repair tissues
7 carbohydrates
8 keep your heart pumping efficiently, muscles
9 lung capacity, oxygen
10 vitamins
11 construction of body tissues
12 waste products
13 smoking, alcohol, drugs
14 beans
15 vegetables

Listening Skills 9

6.2 Healthier life

1 to share
2 to gain weight
3 chunky
4 experiences
5 physical activity
6 broke up
7 abandoned
8 workout routine
9 hard
10 skip
11 self-esteem
12 to fit
13 incentive
14 to achieve
15 target weight
16 results
17 encouragement
18 to be committed
19 zelfbeeld
20 confident

6.4 Grammar: Adjectives and Adverbs

1. seriously
2. serious
3. badly
4. bad
5. good
6. well
7. good
8. differently
9. continuously
10. specially

6.6 Anatomy

1. hair
2. fore head
3. nose
4. chin
5. chest
6. stomach
7. thumb
8. arm
9. belly button / navel
10. knee
11. foot
12. ankle
13. thigh
14. heel
15. neck
16. nape of the neck
17. head
18. shoulder blade
19. penis
20. testicles
21. buttocks
22. vagina
23. calf
24. fingers
25. wrist
26. elbow
27. spine
28. armpit
29. waist
30. nipple

6.7 The Plural

1. children
2. men, teeth
3. means
4. scissors, newspapers
5. cats, lives

6 potatoes
7 contents, boxes
8 wives
9 feet
10 countries

6.8 Idioms

1 The committee will present new sanitary measures.
2 They need education about safe sex and use of condoms.
3 Your health is the condition of your body.
4 A new scheme to teach mothers more about nutrition.
5 We are fighting pollution to protect the environment.
6 We need vitamins to remain healthy.
7 An alcoholic is someone who is addicted to alcohol.
8 Passive smoking can increase the risk of lung cancer.
9 Fresh water is water that is suitable for drinking.
10 The poison may be absorbed through the skin.

6.10 State of mind

1. verdrietig –	sad –	mournful
2. blij –	happy –	cheerful
3. teruggetrokken –	withdrawn –	retired
4. somber –	gloomy –	dark
5. boos –	angry –	mad
6. geërgerd –	annoyed –	agitated
7. depressief –	depressed –	low
8. geïrriteerd –	irritated –	edgy
9. bang –	afraid –	scared
10. overstuur –	upset –	shaken

GPSR Compliance

The European Union's (EU) General Product Safety Regulation (GPSR) is a set of rules that requires consumer products to be safe and our obligations to ensure this.

If you have any concerns about our products, you can contact us on

ProductSafety@springernature.com

In case Publisher is established outside the EU, the EU authorized representative is:

Springer Nature Customer Service Center GmbH
Europaplatz 3
69115 Heidelberg, Germany

www.ingramcontent.com/pod-product-compliance
Lightning Source LLC
Chambersburg PA
CBHW081226100426
42871CB00020B/246

9 789031 349876